Applied equine nutrition and training

Applied equine nutrition and training

Equine NUtrition and TRAining COnference
(ENUTRACO) 2015

edited by: Arno Lindner

 Arbeitsgruppe Pferd

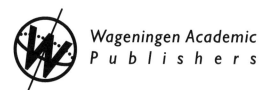

EAN: 9789086862726
e-EAN: 9789086868186
ISBN: 978-90-8686-272-6
e-ISBN: 978-90-8686-818-6
DOI: 10.3920/978-90-8686-818-6

First published, 2015

© Wageningen Academic Publishers
The Netherlands, 2015

Table of contents

Expanded abstracts

Editorial

The Equine NUtrition and TRAining COnference – ENUTRACO – started with the name Equine NUtrition COnference – ENUCO – in 2005 in Hanover, Germany. Already in 2007 in Vienna, Austria, the content on training of horses increased markedly despite that the name of the conference continued to be ENUCO. Since, the meetings in Madrid, Spain (2009), Paris, France (2011), and Bonn, Germany (2013) have been more and more dedicated to the subject of training sport horses and were run under the name ENUTRACO. In 2013 the rehabilitation of horses became an important component of the conference. Now, ENUTRACO is hold in Bingen and Waldalgesheim, Germany, and I am very tempted to change next time the name of the event again to reflect the importance of the theme rehabilitation in this event too! Comments are very welcome!

Thank you to all speakers for their work, to Kai Kreling for providing his equine clinic and rehabilitation centre for the conference courses and to all those attending for sharing their expertise!

Wish you health and a good time!

Arno Lindner

Articles

1. How to feed sport horses with roughage only

A. Jansson

Swedish University of Agricultural Sciences, Department of Animal Nutrition and Management, P.O. Box 7024, 750 07 Uppsala, Sweden; anna.jansson@slu.se

Abstract

Performance horses are commonly fed diets including large amounts of starch-rich concentrates despite that there is little scientific evidence that such diets promote performance. In contrast, it is well known that high concentrate diets can cause gastrointestinal problems, stereotypical behaviour and perhaps also musculoskeletal problems. High energy roughage-only diets could be an alternative to high concentrate diets and promote both health and performance in sport horses. This paper reviews the main studies performed on this subject. The studies have focused on performance, digestion, metabolism and fluid balance. It is concluded that diets based on high energy forage are an alternative to conventional high starch diets.

Keywords: concentrate, diet, forage, exercise, performance

Introduction

Horses have evolved as grass eaters. Nevertheless, performance horses are commonly fed diets including large amounts of starch-rich concentrates (Jansson and Harris, 2013). One reason for using high-concentrate diets is simply that the energy density of traditional horse grass forages often does not meet requirements and concentrate supplementation is needed to maintain body condition. There seems also to be a belief among riders and trainers that concentrate is needed for maximal performance. Interestingly, there is little scientific evidence that starch-rich concentrates promote performance but it is well known that high concentrate diets can cause gastrointestinal problems and stereotypical behaviour and perhaps also musculoskeletal problems (McLeay *et al.*, 1999; Valberg, 1998).

A. Lindner (ed.) *Applied equine nutrition and training (ENUTRACO 2015)*
DOI 10.3920/978-90-8686-818-6_1, © Wageningen Academic Publishers 2015

There is therefore a need for studies on alternative feeding strategies that matches the biology of horses. Grass is an obvious first choice of investigation.

Grass is comprised mainly of fibre and grass forage energy content is mainly dependent on the organic matter digestibility. The fibre and organic matter digestibility is affected by botanical maturity at harvest, and the energy content of grass forages cut at an early stage of maturity is high, comparable to that of oats. During the past 10 years we have had the hypothesis that early cut grass forage diets could be an alternative to high concentrate diets and that such diets might even improve performance. As earlier mentioned, this is in contrast with the belief of many practitioners. This believe is probably to some extent based on true observations, i.e. horses have lost body condition and/or increased body weight and gut fill when offered high forage diets. An increase in body weight and exercise heart rate with a high forage-diet is also supported by observations by Ellis *et al.* (2002). However, that study did not include forage with very high digestibility, which is needed to support the energy requirements of for example Standardbred and Thoroughbred horses in training. It is likely that forage with high organic matter digestibility will result in less gut fill and accordingly, less increase in body weight.

Other theoretical concerns with the use of high energy grass forage to sport horses could be high crude protein intake and low glucose uptake. Grass harvested at an early botanical stage of maturity may have crude protein (CP) contents exceeding the requirements of adult horses. Excessive CP intake will increase urea production and accordingly, the production of hydrogen ions and heat, which in theory could have a negative effect on performance. High CP diets have also not been recommended to exercising horses (Meyer, 1987) and they have even been suggested to reduce performance (Glade, 1983). Another issue with high forage diets may be reduced availability of glucose compared with high starch diets. Grass forages generally contain 5-20% of water soluble carbohydrates on a dry matter (DM) basis and assuming a daily DM intake of 10 kg would result in a daily water soluble carbohydrate intake in the range of 500-2,000 g. Oats contain 20-40% starch and with a daily allowance of 6 kg (Jansson and Harris 2013) this alone would provide 1,200-2,400 g. High blood glucose levels and large glycogen stores could have a positive effect on performance (Farris *et al.*, 1998; Lacombe *et al.*, 2001) and low starch diets post-exercise could potentially impair recovery of muscle glycogen stores (Lacombe *et al.*, 2004).

Nevertheless, we have had the hypothesis that high forage diets actually would improve performance rather than the opposite. Training studies on Standardbred and Thoroughbred horses show that increased aerobic energy metabolism and efficient use of glucose are important training effects (Hinchcliff *et al.*, 2008) and therefore crucial for good performance. Interestingly, similar adaptations have been observed in horses adapted to high fat (Pagan *et al.*, 2002) or high fibre diets (Palmgren-Karlsson *et al.*, 2002), indicating that such diets could be beneficial for performance. High fibre diets increase the availability of the volatile fatty acid acetate compared to diets including starch rich concentrates and it could therefore be hypothesised that with a forage-only diet, substrate utilisation during exercise will resemble the metabolism observed by Pagan *et al.* (2002) and Palmgren-Karlsson *et al.* (2002) on high fat and fibre diets. We have addressed all the issues mentioned above in studies during the past years. Specifically, the studies performed have focused on:

- Body weight and metabolic response, both at rest and exercise, to forage-only diets compared with conventional forage-concentrate diets (Connysson *et al.*, 2010; Jansson and Lindberg, 2012).
- Exercise response and fluid and acid balance on forage diets with different CP contents (Connysson *et al.*, 2006).
- Muscle glycogen content on forage-only and conventional diets (Essén-Gustavsson *et al.*, 2010; Jansson and Lindberg, 2012; Ringmark *et al.*, 2012; Ringmark *et al.*, unpublished data).
- Effects of forage preservation method on fluid balance and exercise response (Muhonen *et al.*, 2009b).
- The possibility to get yearling Standardbred horses in condition to race at an age of three on a forage-only diet (Ringmark *et al.*, 2015).
- Effects of a forage-only and a conventional diet on the hindgut ecosystem (Willing *et al.*, 2009).

The aim of this article is to summarise the results and conclusions.

Horses and diets studied

In our studies, Standardbred horses in race training have been used. These horses are known to have very high energy requirements, equal to those of Thoroughbred race horses, and could therefore be considered as a good 'sport horse model'. The horses included in our studies were fed grass forages consisting mainly of timothy and meadow fescue. The energy content of the forages was always analysed prior to feeding and was >10 MJ metabolisable energy (ME) (corresponding to >11.5 MJ digestible energy) per kg DM. The forages were also analysed for CP, calcium (Ca), phosphorus (P) and magnesium (Mg) content. In a few cases when feeding growing horses (Ringmark et al., 2015), the diet had to be supplemented with lucerne to meet the CP requirements (according to NRC, 2007) and in another study (Muhonen et al., 2009b) the diet was supplemented with another roughage (molassed sugar beet pulp, 18% of total DM intake) to meet the energy requirements. In almost all cases, supplementation with Ca and P was needed (NRC, 2007) and vitamins and trace minerals were added to ensure that deficiencies did not occur. The dry matter (DM) content of the forages varied between 45 and 85% and all batches were preserved in big bales wrapped in plastic.

Effects on performance, body condition and glycogen stores

It has been shown that the velocity at which Standardbred horses reach plasma lactate concentration 4 mmol/l during an incremental exercise test (V_{La4}) is correlated to true race performance (Leleu et al. 2005), i.e. the higher the V_{La4} the better the performance. We have observed that the plasma lactate concentration after an incremental exercise was lower on a forage-only diet compared to a traditional diet and also that there was a tendency for higher V_{La4} (Jansson and Lindberg, 2012). In the same study, plasma glucose concentration and venous pH were also higher in connection with exercise on the forage-only diet. High blood glucose levels might improve performance (Farris et al. 1998) and increased venous pH might partly counteract the exercise-induced acidosis typical, and probably limiting, for high intensity exercise. We have also shown that it is possible to get yearling Standardbred horses in condition to race and win at the age of three on a forage-only diet (Ringmark, 2014; Ringmark et al., 2015).

Body condition is also of importance for performance (Kearns *et al.,* 2002; Leleu and Cotrel, 2006). In our studies, body condition has been stable and around 5 (Henneke *et al.,* 1983) in most individuals when fed a forage-only diet. However, 10.2 MJ ME/kg DM appears to be too low to avoid loss of body condition in some individuals.

Low muscle glycogen stores might impair performance (Lacombe *et al.,* 2001). In Standardbred yearlings in training fed forage-only diets, glycogen content was similar or higher than earlier reported in horses in conventional training (Ringmark *et al.,* 2013). Also, in the same horses at the age of two and three, glycogen levels at rest where high (590-620 mmol/kg dry weight) and comparable with other observations on horses fed conventional diets (Ringmark, 2014). In the study by Jansson and Lindberg (2012), resting muscle glycogen content was slightly lower (-13%) on a forage-only diet than on a high concentrate diet, but any effect on true performance of this small reduction remains to be proven. High forage CP content may support high glycogen levels and a significant difference (630 vs 550 mmol/kg dry weight) has been observed in a study comparing forage with 17 and 13% CP (Essén-Gustavsson *et al.,* 2010).

Effects on metabolism and hindgut microflora

In horses fed a forage-only diet, the faecal microflora has been shown to be more stable over time compared to a conventional high starch diet and microbes known to be specialised on starch fermentation is reduced (Willing *et al.,* 2009). The forage-only microbiota included fewer lactobacilli, especially *Streptococcus bovis/equinus,* compared to the traditional diet and *Lactobacillus ruminis* was only found in horses on a high concentrate diet, but not in the same horses on a forage-only diet.

As a result of the presence of a microbiota adapted to fibre fermentation and the comparatively low glucose uptake on a forage-only diet, the plasma acetate availability increases and the insulin response decreases compared with a high concentrate diet (Connysson *et al.,* 2010; Jansson and Lindberg, 2012). Insulin is a potent inhibitor of lipolysis and fatty acid oxidation and the low insulin response on the forage-only diet may therefore increase non-esterified fatty acid availability (Jansson and Lindberg, 2012) and lipid oxidation during exercise. This could imply less reliance on carbohydrate stores for energy transduction and could also be a trigger for improving aerobic energy turn-over. The latter is supported by the reduced lactate response observed on the forage-only diet (Jansson and Lindberg, 2012).

The physiological response to high intensity exercise was not significantly altered in horses fed forages with two different CP contents (17 or 13% of DM; Connysson *et al.,* 2006), but venous pH was numerically lower on the high CP diet. We have observed no effects of forage preservation method (hay, haylage and silage) on the acute exercise response, but digestibility was higher for silage than hay (Muhonen *et al.,* 2009b). However, preservation method and CP intake both affected fluid balance. Silage and high CP intake induced higher estimated evaporative losses, which might be important to consider in horses transported long distances, performing endurance-like exercise and in hot climates.

Effects on growth and body weight in adults

For horses that are supposed to compete successfully at an early age it is important that the diet supports both growth potential and exercise requirements. We have observed no adverse effect on growth in horses fed a forage-only diet. In contrast, growth rate has been high and mature body weight (BW) reached before the age of 36 months (Ringmark, 2014; Ringmark *et al.,* 2012).

In adult horses, our studies have shown that BW might increase with a forage-only diet compared with a high concentrate diet but the increase is less than 1% and only significant with repeated measurements over several days. In situations where horses were transported, the weight increase disappeared, probably through defecation. In addition, our data show that exercise heart rate is not increased by a forage-only diet (Connysson *et al.,* unpublished data; Jansson and Lindberg, 2012). Altogether this implies that BW is not an issue for sport horses on a forage-only diet. Some trainer associate forage diets with a 'big belly' but we have made no such observations.

An increase in BW may be due to increased gastrointestinal fill with organic matter and water, since some fibres have high water-holding capacity. Interestingly, we have found that basal plasma volume can be maintained longer during feed deprivation on a forage-only diet than a high concentrate diet (Connysson *et al.*, 2010). Low feed intake is not uncommon prior to competitions and forage-only diet could therefore be beneficial for performance.

Conclusions and application in practice

The observations we have made show that diets based on high energy forage are an alternative to conventional high starch diets. Forage-based diets could support better health and welfare and seem not to be a limitation to performance. However, the forages used must be analysed and lack of nutrients, i.e. protein, Ca, P, Mg and Na supplemented. It is possible that supplementation with vitamin E and trace minerals also is necessary. Maximal voluntary feed intake appears to be 2-2.5% of BW and an energy content of 10.2 MJ ME/kg DM appears to be too low to avoid loss of body condition in some individuals. We therefore recommend that the energy content should not be lower than 10.5 MJ ME/kg DM in sport horses in heavy training (Table 1). However, horses offered excessive amounts of forage may select the most digestible parts, thereby achieving higher energy intake than estimated from

Table 1. Guidelines for the energy and crude protein content of forages suitable for exercising horses.[a,b]

	Energy content (MJ DE/kg DM)	Ratio CP/MJ (g CP/MJ)	Energy content (MJ ME/kg DM)	Ratio digestible CP/MJ (g digestible CP/MJ)
Growing horses (16-36 months)	>10.5[c]	>10	>9[c]	>6
Adult horses in heavy training and competition	>10.5[c]	>7[d]	>9[c]	>5[d]
Other adult horses	7.5-9.5	>7	6.5-9	>5

[a] CP = crude protein; DE = digestible energy; ME = metabolisable energy; DM = dry matter.

[b] If these guidelines are applied, the need for supplementation with concentrates will be limited. Observe that the dark and light grey areas show the same information, but use different units.

[c] If horses are to maintain condition on forage only, >12 MJ DE and >10.5 MJ ME is required.

[d] Excessive (>8 g CP/MJ DE and >7 g digestible CP/MJ ME) crude protein intake prior to exercise may not be optimal for performance, but could be beneficial during recovery.

feed analysis (Jansson and Lindberg, 2012). If body condition is low, an energy supplement should be provided. In young horses in training kept in a free range system, three but not two, feeding stations (big bales) seem to be enough to maintain body condition in 16 individuals. Feed intake is also affected by forage palatability and maybe even small variations in feed hygiene (Jansson, 2013). Rapid changes between forage batches can affect faecal composition (for example pH, water and CP content) and microflora (Connysson *et al.*, 2006; Muhonen *et al.*, 2009a). Changes should therefore be made over several days or weeks in order to minimise the risk of gastrointestinal disturbances.

Acknowledgements

Thanks to the Swedish Trotting Association, Swedish Horse Racing Totalisator Board, The Swedish Horse Council Foundation, Stiftelsen Svensk Hästforskning, The National Centre for Trotting Education at Wången, Sweden and Trioplast AB for financial support of the studies.

References

Connysson, M., Muhonen, S., Lindberg, J.E., Essén-Gustavsson, B., Nyman, G., Nostell, K. and Jansson, A., 2006. Effects on exercise response, fluid and acid-base balance of protein intake from forage-only diets in Standardbred horses. Equine Veterinary Journal 36: 648-653.

Connysson, M., Essén-Gustavsson, B., Lindberg, J.E. and Jansson, A., 2010. Effects of feed deprivation on Standardbred horses in training fed a forage-only diet and a 50:50 forage-oats diet. Equine Veterinary Journal Suppl. 38: 335-340.

Ellis, J.M., Hollands, T. and Allen, D.E., 2002. Effect of forage intake on bodyweight and performance. Equine Veterinary Journal Suppl. 34: 66-70.

Essén-Gustavsson, B., Connysson, M. and Jansson, A. 2010. Effects of crude protein intake from forage-only diets on muscle amino acids and glycogen levels in horses in training. Equine Veterinary Journal Suppl. 38: 341-346.

Farris, J.W., Hinchcliff, K.W., McKeever, K.H., Lamb, D.R. and Thomson, D.L., 1998. Effects of tryptophan and of glucose on exercise capacity of horses. Journal of Applied Physiology 85: 807-816.

Glade, M.J., 1983. Nutrition and performance of racing Thoroughbreds. Equine Veterinary Journal 15: 31-36.

Henneke, D.R., Potter, G.D., Kreider, J.L. and Yeates, B.F., 1983. Relationship between condition score, physical measurements and body-fat percentage in mares. Equine Veterinary Journal 15: 371-372.

Hinchcliff, K.W., Geor, R.J. and Kaneps, A.J., 2008. Equine Exercise Physiology. Saunders Elsevier, Edinburgh, UK.

Jansson, A., 2013. Forage energy and nutrient content – possibilities and limitations for the athletic horses. In: Proceedings of the 4th Nordic Feed Science Conference, 12-13 June; Uppsala, Sweden, 5-9.

Jansson, A. and Harris, P., 2013. A bibliometric review on nutrition of the exercising horse from 1970 to 2010. Comparative Exercise Physiology 9: 169-180.

Jansson, A. and Lindberg, J.E., 2012. A forage-only diet alters the metabolic response of horses in training. Animal 6: 1939-1946.

Kearns, C.F., McKeever, K.H., Kumagai, K. and Abe, T., 2002. Fat-free mass is related to one-mile race performance in elite standardbred horses. Veterinary Journal 163: 260-266.

Lacombe, V.A., Hinchcliff, K.W., Geor, R.J. and Baskin, C.R., 2001. Muscle glycogen depletion and subsequent replenishment affect anaerobic capacity of horses. Journal of Applied Physiology 91: 1782-1790.

Lacombe, V.A., Hinchcliff, K.W., Kohn, C.W., Devor, S.T. and Taylor, L.E., 2004. Effects of feeding meals with various soluble-carbohydrate content on muscle glycogen synthesis after exercise in horses. American Journal of Veterinary Research 65: 916-923.

Leleu, C., Cotrel, C. and Courouce-Malblanc, A., 2005. Relationships between physiological variables and race performance in French Standardbred trotters. Veterinary Record 156: 339-342.

Leleu, C. and Cotrel, C., 2006. Body composition in young Standardbreds in training: relationships to body condition score, physiological and locomotor variables during exercise. Equine Veterinary Journal 38: 98-101.

McLeay, J.M., Valberg, S.J., Pagan, J.D., Xue, J.L., De La Corte, F.D., Roberts, J., 1999. Effect of diet on Thoroughbred horses with recurrent exertional rhabdomyolysis performing a standardised exercise test. Equine Veterinary Journal 30: 458-462.

Meyer, H., 1987. Feeding of horses for eventing and endurance riding. Futterung von Vielseitigkeits-und Distanzpferden. Praktische Tierarzt 68(2): 16-28.

Muhonen, S., Julliand, V., Lindberg, J. E., Bertilsson, J. and Jansson, A., 2009a. Effects on the equine colon ecosystem of feeding silage or haylage after an abrupt change from hay. Journal of Animal Science 87: 2291-2298.

Muhonen, S., Lindberg, J.E., Bertilsson, J. and Jansson, A., 2009b. Effects on fluid balance and exercise response in Standardbred horses feed silage, haylage and hay. Comparative Exercise Physiology 5: 133-142.

NRC, 2007. National Research Council, Nutrient Requirements of Horses. 6th rev. ed. National Academic Press, Washington, DC, USA.

Pagan, J., Geor, R.J., Harris, P.A., Hoekstra, K., Gardner, S., Hudson, C. and Prince, A., 2002. Effects of fat adaptation on glucose kinetics and substrate oxidation during low-intensity exercise. Equine Veterinary Journal Suppl. 34: 33-38.

Palmgren-Karlsson, C. Lindberg, J.E., Jansson, A. and Essén-Gustavsson, B., 2002. Effect of molassed sugar beet pulp on nutrient utilisation and metabolic parameters during exercise. Equine Veterinary Journal Suppl. 34: 44-49.

Ringmark, S., Roepstorff, L., Essén-Gustavsson, B., Revold, T., Lindholm, A., Hedenström, U., Rundgren, M., Ögren, G. and Jansson, A., 2012. Growth, training response and health in Standardbred yearlings fed a forage-only diet. Animal 7: 746-753.

Ringmark, S., Lindholm, A., Hedenström, U., Lindinger, M., Dahlborn, K., Kvart, C. and Jansson, A., 2015. Reduced high intensity training distance had no effect on V_{La4} but attenuated heart rate response in 2-3-year-old Standardbred horses. Acta Veterinaria Scandinavica 57: 17.

Ringmark, S., 2014. A forage-only diet and reduced high intensity training distance in Standradbred horses. Acta Universitatis Agriculturae Sueciae. Doctoral Thesis 80, Swedish University of Agricultural Sciences, Sweden.

Valberg, S.J., 1998. Exertional rhabdomolysis in the horse. In: Pagan, J.D. (ed.) Advances in Equine Nutrition. Nottingham University Press, Manor Farm, Trumpton, UK, pp. 507-512.

Willing, B., Vörös, S., Roos, S., Jones, A., Jansson, A. and Lindberg, J.E., 2009. Changes in faecal bacteria associated with concentrate and forage-only diets fed to horses in training. Equine Veterinary Journal 41: 908-914.

2. Medicinal plants for animals – a current therapeutic option with long tradition

M. Walkenhorst

Department of Livestock Science, Research Institute for Organic Agriculture, Ackerstrasse 113, 5070 Frick, Switzerland; michael.walkenhorst@fibl.org

Abstract

Phytotherapy – the use of medicinal plants or plants rich in secondary metabolites – holds a large and widely unemployed potential to treat diseased animals or to improve the overall animal health situation. The base of this therapy is the tradition, but there is evidence available of the effects of the plant species specific multi component composition and of plant secondary metabolites. These are reviewed in this article conceding that much more clinical research for the veterinary use of medicinal plants is urgently needed.

Keywords: doping, herbal drugs, horse, mistletoe, phytotherapy, sarcoid, secondary plant metabolites

Coevolution and animal self-medication

The first plants were on our planet some 700 million years ago, long before mammals or even the human race. Since then they have to cope with living conditions, including virus, bacteria, fungi and parasites. Hence, the mechanisms of plants to fight against pathogens or to cooperate with (micro-)organism are based on a hundreds of millions of years old coevolution and 'experience'. As there are still a lot of plants on our planet the plants concept might be successful, even though they never developed an immune system. Later plants 'learned' to deal with larger herbivores, even though they are not able to run (away). This bondage to the growing place has also as a consequence that communication, sexuality and reproduction of plants is dependent on other mechanisms than in animals.

One of the mechanisms which plants developed to deal with these challenges are the so called plant secondary metabolites (PSM). These PSM are very diverse from the chemical point of view and fulfil specific and also very diverse 'jobs' for the plants.

From the viewpoint of our recent mammals, for example horses, even they look back to a coevolution with plants of several millions of years. In consequence they 'learned' to cope with PSM via detoxifying metabolisms like glucoronidation of phenolic molecules in the liver (Baojian *et al.*, 2011). This coevolution goes even so far, that, up to a certain degree, some kind of physiological dependence on PSM develops as it is discussed recently for bitter substances in human nutrition (Drewnowski and Gomez-Carneros, 2000). On the other hand there is a rising number of scientific publications dealing with animal self-medication in primates (Huffman *et al.*, 1997) but also in other animal species. Animals develop in special pathological situations, for example in times with a high parasite burden, a special ingestion behaviour.

History of medicinal plant use

Self-medication with plants is also documented as a human behaviour since human behaviour could be documented. A pollen analysis of an Irakian grave suggests the active use of medicinal plants some 60,000 years ago. Starting with Dioscurides ('*De material medica*') about 2,000 years ago more and more therapeutic uses of plants have been documented in writing in Europe. For a long time no differentiation between human and veterinary medicine was made but as long humans domesticated animals as long they will have treated their animals with plants. Until 1950 medicinal plants were the base of veterinary pharmacotherapy even in central Europe which is well documented in books (Fröhner, 1900) or typoscripts of lectures in veterinary pharmacology (Steck, 1944), but in the last 60 years this knowledge got more and more lost (Löscher *et al.*, 1994).

Current ethnoveterinary research

Medicinal plants are still the base of unbroken traditional therapeutic systems in large parts of the world, for example in Asia. In Europe only very few veterinarians are still familiar with medicinal plants.

In contrast a wide spectrum of medicinal plants and other plants rich in PSM is still used traditionally by farmers to treat different kinds of diseases in livestock (Disler *et al.*, 2014; Mayer *et al.*, 2014; Schmid *et al.*, 2012). In Switzerland, in the frame of an ongoing project, a total of 108 interviews with 137 persons were conducted between 2011-2013. More than 800 use reports based on 109 plant species have been registered; chamomile (*Matricaria chamomilla* L.) and Marigold flowers (*Calendula officinalis* L.) being the most frequently reported for use against skin diseases and wounds as well as diseases of the gastro intestinal tract (Walkenhorst *et al.*, 2014).

In Europe the majority of ethnoveterinary research is from the Mediterranean countries, particularly Italy and Spain (Akerreta *et al.*, 2010; Benítez *et al.*, 2012; Gonzalez *et al.*, 2011; Pieroni *et al.*, 2004, 2006; Viegi *et al.*, 2003). A recent review, based on 75 scientific publications including a total of 2,688 European ethnoveterinary use reports, documents: 'a total of 590 plant species referring to 102 different plant families are reported to be used for animal treatment, with *Asteraceae*, *Fabaceae* and *Lamiaceae* being the most important families' (Mayer *et al.*, 2014).

Recent veterinary challenges: might phytotherapy be an option?

Antimicrobial resistance of pathogens or even apathogenic bacteria are becoming a major concern both in humans and animals (WHO, 2014; Woolhouse *et al.*, 2015). The overuse of antibiotics is the main reason for this.

There is no standard definition of phytotherapy, but the common agreement of different scientific and therapeutic societies is that herbal drugs are based on extracts containing at least a part of the plant species specific combination of PSM and not only one single substance (Meier *et al.*, 2014). Compared to antibiotics (which are in most cases single substances) the extracts from medicinal plants are multi-component compositions and have therefore only a low risk to raise resistances. Several plant extracts affect even biofilms (Wojnicz *et al.*, 2012) or activate the immune system (Schapowal, 2013). A lot of pharmaceutical, pharmacological and human clinical research is available (ESCOP, 2003; Meier *et al.*, 2014) but it is still missing in the field of animal health care and veterinary medicine (Walkenhorst *et al.*, 2014).

Phytotherapy – main fields of application

Due to their missing immunity plants have first of all to defend their surfaces. Maybe in consequence one of their most important therapeutic fields of application are surfaces: skin diseases and wounds, gastrointestinal and respiratory diseases. Some examples of medicinal plants with these uses follow below.

Skin diseases

Only very few different ingredients, almost all are disinfectants or antibiotics, are available in registered veterinary drugs to treat skin diseases and wounds. Particularly in wound healing not only antimicrobial activity is needed but also anti-inflammatory activity or the stimulation of re-epithelization is important. So plants might be here a real option to enlarge the therapeutic spectrum.

Salvia (*Salvia officinalis* L.)

Salvia stands for the classical combination of tannins and essential oils in plants. Tannins denaturise proteins in the wound and seal the injured tissue. Essential oils show antimicrobial properties. As well as for the skin salvia can be used for internal surfaces for example regarding the oral mucosa. Several *in vitro* studies show the antiviral and antibacterial properties of salvia (ESCOP, 2003). A special focus might be the antifungal activity of salvia (ESCOP, 2003) in the future due to the fact that there is only one registered antifungal substance on the market to treat livestock.

Marigold flower (*Calendula officinalis* L.)

Marigold flower is one of the typical drugs to explain the reasonability of phytotherapy. As a whole marigold flower stimulates the fibroplasia, the angiogenesis and shows anti-inflammatory and antibacterial properties (Parente *et al.*, 2012), but none of the single components is able to show these effects alone. Essential oils, triterpene saponines, sesquiterpenoids and sterols are constituents of marigold flower (ESCOP, 2003). Farmers in Switzerland manufacture since generations tincture and ointments to treat wounds and care for skin (Disler *et al.*,

2014; Walkenhorst *et al.*, 2014). Marigold flower is recommended for the treatment of minor wounds and skin inflammation (ESCOP, 2003).

Gastro intestinal tract

Diarrhoea is one of the main reasons for the huge amount of antibiotics which is still used in veterinary medicine. But also obstipation could be cause for a treatment. Furthermore, indigestions and other diseases come along with reduced appetite.

Linseed (*Linum usitatissimum* L.)

To be protected from auto-ingestion intestinal mucosa is coated with mucilage. Even the gastro intestinal tract itself produces these polysaccharids. In case of reduced production of these protecting substances (e.g. in case of gastritis or enteritis) a mucilage based on plants achieve a mitigation. Depending on the target location the mucilage linseed will be given orally already swollen (for gastric problems) or as pure linseed combined with an extra portion of water (enteric problems). The later administration is also an option to treat mild cases of obstipation (ESCOP, 2003).

Black tea (*Camelia sinensis* L.)

Black tea contains tannins. Antidiarrheal properties have been found in several studies (Besra *et al.*, 2003). Caffeine is one of its ingredients and is helpful in the case of lethargic animals. In particular diarrhoea therapy is a good example how easy and practicable medicinal plants can be combined with the standard therapy, which is, first of all, an oral rehydration. Instead of mixing dextrose and minerals just with water it is easy to mix it with an infusion like from black tea or, depending on the symptoms, also from chamomile (anti-inflammatory properties) or caraway (spasmolytic properties).

Wormwood (*Arthemisia absinthium* L.)

Ingestion can be caused by a malsecretion of intestinal enzymes of liver, pancreas and other intestinal glands. Due to their coevolution herbivores are well adapted and maybe even dependent to some bitter substances in their rations. It is well known that bitter receptors are widely spread all over the gastro intestinal tract and even in other tissues. When they are stimulated the secretion and production of digestive excretes raises (ESCOP, 2003). A side effect is the appetizing property of bitter substances. Wormwood is one representative of bitter substances (ESCOP, 2003).

Respiratory tract

Infectious diseases as well as chronic obstructive diseases of the respiratory tract are severe problems in many animal species.

Thyme (*Thymus vulgaris* L.)

Thymol and carvacrol are the major constituents of thyme essential oil (ESCOP, 2003); the bronchodilatating properties have been demonstrated with isolated tracheas of guinea pigs (Boskabady *et al.*, 2006). Thyme extracts show antispasmodic properties in rat tracheal smooth muscle cells and they increase the mucociliary transport in mice (Begrow *et al.*, 2010). Thyme essential oil shows high antimicrobial activities on major pathogens of the respiratory tract (Fabio *et al.*, 2007). The essential oils are well suited for a nearly neglected but still reasonable administration procedure: inhalation. Besides the transport of essential oil directly to the respiratory tract, also water reaches the bronchi and helps there to fluidise tough mucus.

My personal 'starting drug' – chamomile (Matricaria recutita L.)

Chamomile might be one of the most famous European medicinal plants at all and it is recently the most often documented plant species in Swiss ethnoveterinarian research (Walkenhorst *et al.*, 2014). Chamomile could be used as well in gastrointestinal as in skin diseases and in the respiratory tract. The main ingredients of chamomile are essential oils and flavonoids. The essential oils (lipophilic) show anti-inflammatory and the flavonoids (water soluble) spasmolytic activities on smooth muscles (ESCOP, 2003). Depending on the extraction procedure the one or the other property prevails. A tea is beneficial in case of diarrhoea due to its spasmolytic function and inhalation transports the essential oils in the upper respiratory tract to modulate inflammation and reduce the infectious burden.

Equine sarcoid – mistletoe as a therapeutic option

Extracts of *Viscum album* L. (VAE) are widely used as adjuvant in human cancer therapy and cytotoxicity in cancer cell lines have been described recently (Klingbeil *et al.*, 2013). In an prospective, randomised and blinded clinical trial 53 horses with clinical diagnosed equine sarcoids were treated three times weekly for 15 weeks with 1 ml subcutaneous injections of a VAE (Iscador P). No adverse effects could be observed except of a mild oedema at the injection site in about 15% of the treated horses. A complete or partial regression of sarcoids could be observed in 41% of the horses of the VAE group compared to 14% of the control group. This difference was significant ($P < 0.05$; Christen-Clottu *et al.*, 2010).

Current regulatory situation

Veterinary herbal drugs

The EU regulation 37/2010 contains more than 60 different medicinal plant species (EC, 2010) as active substance in livestock (all without a withdrawal period) but the particular regulation regarding the handling of medicinal plants differs widely between countries. Nevertheless European-wide only around 10 registered veterinary drugs solely based on medicinal plants are available. The use of plants as medication for animals in the European Union depends furthermore on their status, and horses could be both: In livestock this particular use is restricted to (depending on possible stricter regulation in some countries) at maximum these 60 plant species but only in cases where a rededication is allowed; in case of companion animals even the whole spectrum of human herbal drugs could be used but also only in cases where rededication is allowed. In Switzerland the use of medicinal plants is allowed and for this a rededication is not claimed but the list of usable plants for livestock contains only around 20 plant species.

Herbal feed additives

There is a large and growing European market for herbal feed additives, in particular for horses, but even the quantity of herbal ingredients varies widely. No regulations exist regarding the content and quality of herbal ingredients. For the user it is nearly impossible to divide between feed additives with high quality ingredients – partly even pharmaceutic quality – and products containing only negligible low doses of herbs. Furthermore these products are normally bought and used directly by the animal keepers with low or even without knowledge regarding potential effects (or side-effects) of the plants contained.

Doping

Diverse and oftentimes changing regulations exist regarding the handling of medicinal plants and plant secondary metabolites as doping substances in different federations (and even regional subunits) of sport horses. Some spectacular cases emerged during the last decades, based on the intended or even accidental 'use' of medicinal plants. Valerian, willow (salicylate) and chillies (capsaicin) were recently banned. The doping relevance of other plants like coffee, cacao, black tea, devils claw (*Harpagophytum procumbens* D.C.), ginger, ginseng, and kava is unclear. The use of arnica, olibanum, comfrey and rose hip – all of them show slight anti-inflammatory properties – seems to be save at the moment.

Conclusions

Phytotherapy – the use of medicinal plants or plants rich in secondary metabolites – holds a large and widely unemployed potential to treat diseased animals or to improve the overall animal health situation. The base of this therapy is the tradition, but there is more and more evidence available of the effects of the plant species specific multi component composition and of plant secondary metabolites. More clinical research for the veterinary use of medicinal plants is urgently needed, but for some plants there is already enough evidence available to start to gain own experiences.

References

Akerreta, S., Calvo, M.I. and Cavero, R.Y., 2010. Ethnoveterinary knowledge in Navarra (Iberian Peninsula). Journal of Ethnopharmacology 130: 369-378.

Baojian, W., Kaustubh, K., Sumit, B., Shuxing, Z., and Hu, M., 2011. First-pass metabolism via UDP-glucuronosyltransferase: a barrier to oral bioavailability of phenolics. Journal of Pharmaceutical Sciences 100: 3655-3681.

Begrow, F., Engelbertz, J., Feistel, B., Lehnfeld, R., Bauer, K. and Verspohl, E.J., 2010. Impact of thymol in thyme extracts on their antispasmodic action and ciliary clearance. Planta Medica 76: 311-318.

Benítez, G., González-Tejero, M.R. and Molero-Mesa, J., 2012. Knowledge of ethnoveterinary medicine in the Province of Granada, Andalusia, Spain. Journal of Ethnopharmacology 139: 429-439.

Besra, S., Gomes, A., Ganguly, D. and Vedasiromoni, J., 2003. Antidiarrhoeal activity of hot water extract of black tea (*Camellia sinensis*). Phytotherapy Research 17: 380-384.

Boskabady, M.H., Aslani, M.R. and Kiani, S., 2006. Relaxant effect of *Thymus vulgaris* on guinea-pig tracheal chains and its possible mechanism(s). Phytotherapy Research 20: 28-33.

Christen-Clottu, O., Klocke, P., Burger, D., Straub R. and Gerber, V., 2010. Treatment of clinically diagnosed equine sarcoid with a mistletoe extract (*Viscum album austriacus*). Journal of Veterinary Internal Medicine 24: 1483-1489.

Disler, M., Ivemeyer, S., Hamburger, M., Vogl, C., Tesic, A., Klarer, F., Meier, B. and Walkenhorst, M., 2014. Ethnoveterinary herbal remedies used by farmers in four north-eastern Swiss cantons (St. Gallen, Thurgau, Appenzell Innerrhoden and Appenzell Ausserrhoden). Journal of Ethnobiology and Ethnomedicine 10: 32.

Drewnowski, A., and Gomez-Carneros, C., 2000. Bitter taste, phytonutrients, and the consumer: a review. American Journal of Clinical Nutrition 72: 1424-1435.

European Scientific Cooperative on Phytotherapy (ESCOP), 2003. ESCOP Monographs, 2nd ed. Georg Thieme Verlag, Stuttgart, Germany.

European Commission (EC), 2010. Commission Regulation (EU) No 37/2010 of 22 December 2009 on pharmacologically active substances and their classification regarding maximum residue limits in foodstuffs of animal origin. Official Journal European Union L15: 1-72.

Fabio, A., Cermelli, C., Fabio, G., Nicoletti, P. and Quaglio, P., 2007. Screening of the antibacterial effects of a variety of essential oils on microorganisms responsible for respiratory infections. Phytotherapeutic Research 21: 374-387.

Fröhner, E., 1900. Lehrbuch der Arzneimittellehre für Thierärtze, 5th ed. Ferdinand Enke, Stuttgart, Germany.

Gonzalez, J.A., Garcia-Barriuso, M. and Amich, F., 2011. Ethnoveterinary medicine in the Arribes del Duero, western Spain. Veterinary Research Communications 35: 283-310.

Huffman, M.A., Gotoh, S., Turner, A.L., Hamai, M. and Yoshida, K., 1997. Seasonal trends in intestinal nematode infection and medicinal plant use among chimpanzees in the Mahale Mountains, Tanzania. Primates 38: 111-125.

Klingbeil, M.F., Xavier, F.C., Sardinha, L.R., Severino, P., Mathor, M.B., Rodrigues, R.V., and Pinto Jr., D.S., 2013. Cytotoxic effects of mistletoe (*Viscum album* L.) in head and neck squamous cell carcinoma cell lines. Oncology Reports 30: 2316-2322.

Löscher, W., Ungemach, F.R. and Kroker, R., 1994. Grundlagen der Pharmakotherapie bei Haus- und Nutztieren. In: W. Löscher, F.R. Ungemach and R. Kroker (eds.), Grundlagen der Pharmakotherapie bei Haus- und Nutztieren. Verlag Paul Parey, Berlin, Germany, pp. 400-401.

Mayer, M., Vogl, C.R., Amorena, M., Hamburger, M. and Walkenhorst, M., 2014. Treatment of organic livestock with medicinal plants: a systematic review of European ethnoveterinary research. Forschende Komplementmedizin 21: 375-386.

Meier, B., Saller, R. and Walkenhorst, M. (eds.), 2014. Internationale Tagung Phytotherapie 2014, Klinik und Praxis, 29. Schweizerische Jahrestagung für Phytotherapie, 18-21 June 2014, Winterthur, Referate und Poster Abstracts. Forschende Komplementärmedizin 21 (Suppl. 1).

Parente, L.M.L., De Souza Jr., R.L., Faustino L.M.T., Vinaud, M.C., De Paula, J.R. and Paulo, N.M., 2012. Wound healing and anti-inflammatory effect in animal models of *Calendula officinalis* L. growing in Brazil. Evidence-Based Complementary and Alternative Medicine 2012: 375671.

Pieroni, A., Giusti, M., De Pasquale, C., Lenzarini, C., Censorii, E., Gonzales-Tejero, M., Sanchez-Rojas, C., Ramiro-Gutierrez, J., Skoula, M., Johnson, C., Sarpaki, A., Della, A., Paraskeva-Hadijchambi, D., Hadjichambis, A., Hmamouchi, M., El-Jorhi, S., El-Demerdash, M., El-Zayat, M., Al-Shahaby, O., Houmani, Z. and Scherazed, M., 2006. Circum-Mediterranean cultural heritage and medicinal plant uses in traditional animal healthcare: a field survey in eight selected areas within the RUBIA project. Journal of Ethnobiology and Ethnomedicine 2: 1-16.

Pieroni, A., Howard, P., Volpato, G. and Santoro, R., 2004. Natural remedies and nutraceuticals used in ethnoveterinary practices in inland southern Italy. Veterinary Research Communications 28: 55-80.

Schapowal, A., 2013. Efficacy and safety of Echinaforce® in respiratory tract infections. Wiener Medizinische Wochenschrift 163: 102-105.

Schmid, K., Ivemeyer, S., Hamburger, M., Vogl, C., Klarer, F., Meier, B. and Walkenhorst, M., 2012. Traditional use of herbal remedies in livestock by farmers in three Swiss cantons (Aargau, Zurich and Schaffhausen). Forschende Komplementärmedizin 19: 125-136.

Steck, W., 1944. Pharmakologie. Typoskript erstellt von Gross, R., Bern (Kopie im Archiv der Schweizerischen Vereinigung für Geschichte der Veterinärmedizin).

Viegi, L., Pieroni, A., Guarrera, P. and Vangelisti, R., 2003. A review of plants used in folk veterinary medicine in Italy as basis for a databank. Journal Ethnopharmacology 89: 221-244.

Walkenhorst, M., Vogl, C., Vogl-Lukasser, B., Vollstedt, S., Brendieck-Worm, C., Ivemeyer, S., Klarer, F., Meier, B., Schmid, K., Disler, M., Bischoff, T., Hamburger, M., Häsler, S. and Stöger, E., 2014. Zwischen Empirie und Evident – (Re) Aktivierung der Veterinärphytotherapie at Internationale Tagung Phytotherapie 2014, Klinik und Praxis: 29. Schweizerische Jahrestagung für Phytotherapie, 18-21 June 2014, Winterthur. Forschende Komplementärmedizin / Research in Complementary Medicine 21(Suppl. 1): 1-70.

World Health Organization (WHO), 2014. Antimicrobial resistance: global report on surveillance 2014. WHO, Geneva, Switzerland. Available at: http://tinyurl.com/oe9v8ma.

Wojnicz, D., Kucharska, A.Z., Sokól-Letowska, A., Kicia, M. and Tichaczek-Goska, D., 2012. Medicinal plants extracts affect virulence factors expression a biofilm formation by uropathogenic *Escherichia coli*. Urological Research 40: 683-697.

Woolhouse, M., Ward, M., van Bunnik, B. and Farrar, J., 2015. Antimicrobial resistance in humans, livestock and the wider environment. Philosophical Transactions Royal Society London B Biological Sciences 370: 1670.

3. Equine immunology and phytogenic drugs: possibilities and limitations

S. Vollstedt

Praxis für Traditionelle Chinesische Pferdemedizin, Hauptstraße 53, 25335 Bokholdt-Hanredder, Germany; tcpm@svollstedt.com

Abstract

The potential effect of herbs to treat lung, skin and gastrointestinal pathologies in horses is discussed. For lung pathologies effects of food supplementation with garlic, aniseed, fennel, licorice, thyme and hyssop have been found. A preparation of yellow gentian, garden sorrel, cowslip, verbena and common elder rendered recurrent airway obstruction affected horses less sensitive to histamine. For skin conditions flax seed and heartsease have a positive effect when fed on a regular basis. *Aloe vera*, along with chrysanthemum, relieves symptoms of dermatitis. Chamomile is one of the oldest known herbs with its anti-inflammatory properties. To manage gastrointestinal disturbances flax seed again is an important resource to support the symbiota. Fenugreek seed is also able to affect the microbiota stabilizing the immune system and *Silybum marianum* can also influence the gut to become healthy.

Keywords: herbs, horse, pathology, rehabilitation, treatment

Introduction

An immune response is an interaction between highly specialized cells with a strict order for how information is passed on. These cells are able to differentiate between self and non-self as well as between pathogenic and non-pathogenic. Therefore, the immune system is always active and examines every particle invading the body (Murphy *et al.*, 2008).

A. Lindner (ed.) *Applied equine nutrition and training (ENUTRACO 2015)*
DOI 10.3920/978-90-8686-818-6_3, © Wageningen Academic Publishers 2015

Wherever there is contact between the environment and the body, as in the lung, the gut or the bladder, specialized dendritic cells (DCs) are scanning for invaders. These cells are also called sentinel cells because they have the ability to distinguish between self and non-self as well as pathogenic and non-pathogenic and alarm the rest of the immune cells that something is happening (Murphy *et al.*, 2008).

Pathogen-associated molecular patterns (PAMPs) on pathogenic microbes are recognized by pattern recognition receptors (PRRs) of the DCs. In particular Toll-like receptors (TLRs) are known to confer information of the pathogen to the DC and induce the release of cytokines to initiate an immune response. With different sets of receptors DC are able to gain information of the nature of the pathogen. They can distinguish between intracellular or extracellular, between bacteria, virus or parasite and if there is single or double stranded DNA or RNA. Thus it enables the DC to activate specific cells, which are needed to control the invasion of the body (Shortman and Naik, 2007).

The immune mechanisms between pathogens differ. Intracellular bacteria require a cellular immune response because the pathogens are mainly found inside host cells and these need to be taken care of as well. On the other hand the humoral immune response is efficient during an extracellular bacterial infection because the pathogens are mainly outside of host cells. Therefore, the immune response can be skewed to either cellular or humoral. Once one of them is initiated there is a restriction on the other one (Shortman and Naik, 2007).

The lung

As long as the environment of a horse consists of a normal load of pathogens the immune system is able to control infections. However, nowadays a lot of horses are housed indoors and do not live in their natural environment. Exposure to dust and fungi is increased and the immune system is overwhelmed with particles that are harmful to the animal (Lanz *et al.*, 2013).

Exposure to dust and high concentrations of fungi have a severe impact on the immune response that can lead to serious harm elicited by the immune cells. It has been shown that DCs produce high amounts of interleukin (IL)-4 which lead to the activation of the humoral pathway with an increase of the neutrophil percentage. On the other hand, especially at a later time point, DC also start to produce high amounts of IL-12 to activate the cellular immune response with an increase of natural killer cells (NK cells), macrophages and cytotoxic T lymphocytes (CTL). Because they are part of the cellular arm, host cells get damaged resulting in bronchiolitis and emphysema (Ainsworth *et al.*, 2003).

In the lung of horses with recurrent airway obstruction (RAO) there is an increase of neutrophilic and basophilic granulocytes as well as mast cells. Cytokines like IL-1b and IL-8 are elevated which attract the aforementioned cells. DCs also produce IL-4 for the initiation of the humoral immune response and elevated immunoglobulin E (IgE), as well as IL-12 and interferon gamma (IFN-γ) for the cellular immune response (Lavoie-Lamoureux *et al.*, 2010).

Inhalation is a long standing therapy in horses affected with lung problems. Eucalyptus oil has been shown to be very effective in reducing the elevated level of IL-4 and to inhibit over-activated macrophages in the lung (Sadlon and Lamson, 2010). One of the active substances is believed to be the monoterpene 1,8-cineol, which is present in eucalyptus oil in high amounts (Juergens, 2014).

Food supplementation with garlic (*Allium sativum*), aniseed (*Pimpinella anisum*), fennel (*Foeniculum vulgare*), licorice (*Glycirrhizae glabra*), thyme (*Thymus vulgaris*) and hyssop (*Hyssopus officinalis*) were shown to decrease the respiratory rate and to increase the ratio of macrophages in a humoral setting, thus, benefitting the horse's condition (Pearson *et al.*, 2014). Although it should be mentioned that abuse of licorice has side effects similar to an overdose of mineralo-corticoids (Omar *et al.*, 2012) and that high doses of garlic lead to anaemia with Heinz bodies (Pearson *et al.*, 2005). Therefore, these two herbs should not be fed on a regular basis, even when the horse suffers from RAO.

A preparation of yellow gentian (*Gentiana lutea*), garden sorrel (*Rumex acetosa*), cowslip (*Primula veris*), verbena (*Verbena vervain*) and common elder (*Sambucus nigra*) administered to horses rendered RAO affected horses less sensitive to histamine (Anour *et al.*, 2005).

Another herbal composite containing extract of thyme (*Thymus vulgaris*) and primula (*P. veris*) decreased the pulmonary pressure and airway resistance but did not improve the clinical symptoms (Van den Hoven *et al.*, 2003).

Omega-3 unsaturated fatty acids (Ω-3 PUFA) were also shown to influence the composition of immune cells in the horse (Khol-Parisini *et al.*, 2007) and led to an improvement of clinical symptoms in horses suffering from RAO (Nogradi *et al.*, 2014). In Traditional Chinese Veterinary Medicine a recipe called Bai He Gu Jin Tang is used successfully for treatment of RAO in horses (Weerapongse, 2006).

Although there seem to be promising herbal remedies and recipes, the focus should be on the management of the horse. It is more important to reduce exposure to dust with high quality food and taking horses out of the indoor housing than to treat the resulting disease.

The skin

Equine eczema has been a problem found mainly in Icelandic ponies for years but, nowadays, it occurs in many other breeds as well. Eczema and dermatitis are allergic reactions to mosquitoes, food, and environmental burdens and they show similar deviations of the immune system as in the lung, such as elevated levels of IgE, mast cells, and basophils found in the lesions (Wagner *et al.*, 2006). Skin problems are extremely difficult to treat, however, it seems that flax seed has a positive effect when fed on a regular basis (O'Neill *et al.*, 2002). It influences the macrophages activity and the synthesis of eicosanoids (Henry *et al.*, 1990) which are derived from Ω-3 PUFA. Heartsease (*Viola tricolore*) is a traditional herb for skin problems that leads to a decrease in the amount of tumour necrosis factor alpha (TNF-α) and IFN-γ in the skin (Hellinger *et al.*, 2014).

Aloe vera, along with chrysanthemum, relieves symptoms of dermatitis both orally and topically (Feily and Namazi, 2009; Man *et al.*, 2012). One of the oldest herbal remedies is chamomile with its anti-inflammatory properties (Srivasta *et al.*, 2010). In addition feverfew, liquorice, and turmeric also show promising results when used for skin problems.

The gut

The gut is one of the biggest immunological organs because here the immune cells learn how to differentiate between the pathogenic bacteria from the non-pathogenic ones (Min *et al.*, 2015). The microbiota has evolved within the gut since millions of years and is an important source of nutrition (Costa *et al.*, 2012). Immune cells from the gut are found in the rest of the body. Herbs that promote the physiological composition of the microbiota are of great value for a healthy gut. Flax seed again is an important resource to support this symbiotic relationship. Fenugreek seed (*Trigonella foenum-graecum*) is also able to affect the microbiota in a positive way by stabilizing the immune system (Zentek *et al.*, 2013). *Silybum marianum* is known to be a potent liver-related herb, but there are hints that it can also influence the gut to become healthy (Evren *et al.*, 2015).

These herbal remedies are very valuable for the equine intestine and they should be used more often even prophylactically. However, if the horse fodder is at fault and the diet lacks the high fibre intake that horses need, they will not be able to cure an abnormal gut flora. With herbal medicine it is possible to treat conditions, where conventional medicine is limited, but it cannot treat bad care management.

References

Ainsworth, D.M., Gruenig, G., Marychak, M.B., Young, J., Wagner, B., Erb, H.N. and Antczak, D.F., 2003. Recurrent airway obstruction (RAO) in horses is characterized by IFN-gamma and IL-8 production in bronchoalveolar lavage cells. Veterinary Immunology Immunopathology 96: 83-91.

Anour, R., Leinker, S. and Van den Hoven, R., 2005. Improvement of the lung function of horses with heaves by treatment with a botanical preparation for 14 days. Veterinary Record 157: 733-736.

Costa, M.C. and Weese, J.S., 2012. The equine intestinal microbiome. Animal Health Research Review 13: 121-128.

Evren, E. and Yurtcu, E., 2015. *In vitro* effects on biofilm viability and antibacterial and antiadherent activities of silymarin. Folia Microbiologica 4: 351-356.

Feily, A. and Namazi, M.R., 2009. *Aloe vera* in dermatology: a brief review. Fiornale Italiano di Deratologia e Venereologia 144: 85-91.

Hellinger, R., Koehback, J., Fedchuk, H., Sauer, B., Huber, R., Gruber, C.W. and Gruendemann, C., 2014. Immunosuppresive activity of an aqueous *Viola tricolor* herbal extract. Journal of Ehnopharmacology 151: 299-306.

Henry, M.M., Moore, J.N., Feldman, E.B., Fischer J.K. and Russell, B., 1990. Effect of dietary alpha-linolenic acid on equine monocyte procoagulatent activity and eicosanoid synthesis. Circulatory Shock 32: 620-625.

Juergens, U.R., 2014. Anti-inflammatory properties of the monoterpene 1.8-cineole: current evidence for co-medication in inflammatory airway diseases. Drug Research 64: 638-646.

Khol-Parisini, A., Van den Hoven, R., Leinker, S., Hulan, H.W. and Zentek, J., 2007. Effects of feeding sunflower oil or seal blubber oil to horses with recurrent airway obstruction. Canadian Journal Veterinary Research 71: 59-65.

Lanz, S., Gerber, V., Marti, E., Rettmer, H., Klukowska-Rötzler, J., Gottstein, B., Matthews, J.B., Pirie, S. and Hamza, E., 2013. Effect of hay dust extract and cyathostomin antigen stimulation on cytokine expression by PBMC in horses with recurrent airway obstruction. Veterinary Immunology Immunopathology 155: 229-237.

Lavoie-Lamoureux, A., Moran, K., Beauchamp, G., Mauel, S., Steinback, F., Lefebvre-Lavoie, J., Martin, J.G. and Lavoie, J.P., 2010. IL-4 activates equine neutrophils and induces a mixed inflammatory cytokine expression profile with enhanced neutrophil chemotactic mediator release *ex vivo*. American Journal Physiology Lung Cellular Molecular Physiology 299: L472-482.

Man, M.Q., Hupe, M., Sun, R., Man, G., Mauro, T.M. and Elias, P.M., 2012. Topical apigenin alleviates cutaneous inflammation in murine models. Evidence Based Complementary Alternative Medicine 2012: 912028.

Min, Y.W. and Rhee, P.L., 2015. The role of microbiota on the gut immunology. Clinical Therapeutics 37: 968-975.

Murphy, K., Travers, P. and Walport, M., 2008. Janeways Immunobiology, 7th ed. Garland Science, New York, NY, USA.

Nogradi, N., Couetil, L.L., Messick, J., Stochelski, M.A. and Burgess, J.R., 2015. Omega-3 fatty acid supplementation provides an additional benefit to a low-dust diet in the management of horses with chronic lower airway inflammatory disease. Journal Veterinary Internal Medicine 29: 299-306.

Omar, H.R., Komarova, I., El-Ghonemi, M., Fathy, A., Rashad, R., Abdelmalak, H.D., Yerramadha, M.R., Ali, Y., Helal, E. and Camporesi, E.M., 2012. Licorice abuse: time to send a warning message. Therapeutic Advances in Endocrinology and Metabolism 3: 125-138.

O'Neil, W., McKee, S. and Clarke, AF., 2002. Flaxseed (*Linum usitassimum*) supplementation associated with reduced skin test lesional area in horses with Culicoides hypersensitivity. Canadian Journal of Veterinary Research 66: 272-277.

Pearson, W., Boermans, H.J., Bettger, W.J., McBride, B.W. and Lindinger, M.I., 2005. Association of maximum voluntary dietary intake of freeze-dried garlic with Heinz body anemia in horses. American Journal Veterinary Research 66: 457-465.

Pearson, W., Charch, A., Brewer, D. and Clarke, A.F., 2007. Pilot study investigating the ability of an herbal composite to alleviate clinical signs of respiratory dysfunction inhorses with recurrent airway obstruction. Canadian Journal of Veterinary Research 71: 145-151.

Sadlon, A.E. and Lamson, D.W., 2010. Immune-modifying and antimicrobial effects of *Eucalyptus* oil and simple inhalation devices. Alternative Medicine Review 15: 33-47.

Shortman, K. and Naik, S.H., 2007. Steady-state and inflammatory dendritic-cell development. Nature Reviews Immunology 7: 19-30.

Srivasta, J.K., Shankar, E. and Gupta, S., 2010. Chamomile: A herbal medicine of the past with bright future. Molecular Medicine Reports 3: 895-901.

Van den Hoven, R., Zappe, H., Zitterl-Eglseer, K., Jugi, M. and Franz, C., 2003. Study of the effect of Bronchipret on the lung function of five Austria saddle horses suffering recurrent airway obstruction (heaves). Veterinary Record 152: 555-557.

Wagner, B., Miller, W.H., Morgan, E.E., Hillegas, J.M., Erb, H.N., Leibold, W. and Antczak, D.F., 2006. IgE and IgG antibodies in skin allergy of the horse. Veterinary Research 37:813-825.

Weerapongse, T., 2006. Clinical management of equine recurrent airway obstruction with a combination of electroacupuncture and Chinese herbal therapy. American Journal of Traditional Chinese Veterinary Medicine 1: 39-42.

Zentek, J., Gaertner, S., Tedin, L., Maenner, K., Mader, A. and Vahjen, W., 2013. Fenugreek seed affects intestinal microbiota and immunological variables in piglets after weaning. British Journal of Nutrition 109: 859-866.

4. Mycotoxicoses in horses: toxins, occurrence in feed, and the search for markers of exposure

M. Gross[1]*, J.I. Bauer[1], S. Wegner[1], K. Friedrich[1], M. Machnik[2] and E. Usleber[1]

[1]Chair of Dairy Sciences, Institute of Veterinary Food Science, Veterinary Faculty, Justus-Liebig-University, Ludwigstr. 21, 35390 Giessen, Germany; [2]Deutsche Sporthochschule Köln, Institute of Biochemistry, Am Sportpark Müngersdorf 6, 50933 Köln, Germany; madeleine.gross@vetmed.uni-giessen.de

Abstract

Infestation with fungi of plants used for animal feeding, and production of mycotoxins by these fungi either pre- or postharvest are a common occurrence worldwide. Adverse effects of these mycotoxins on the performance and health of livestock have been extensively studied. However, compared to other domesticated species, relatively few information is available concerning the practical relevance of mycotoxins in equine species, most notably in Middle Europe. There are several unique adverse reactions of horses towards dietary mycotoxins, with equine leukoencephalomalacia caused by fumonisins being the most notorious example. On a worldwide basis, other relevant clinical aspects of equine mycotoxicoses include neurotoxic, vasoactive or reproductive effects by ergot alkaloids and tremorgenic endophyte toxins. The mycotoxins may be ingested via pasture/hay, commercial feed preparations or plant material used as bedding. Therefore, feed control for mycotoxins is a necessary task, but it does not guarantee complete avoidance of mycotoxins. A practicable means to check the overall exposure level would be helpful, both in case of clinical disease, and to avoid subclinical or chronic effects of mycotoxins. In this paper, we address some of the most relevant mycotoxins, discuss potential target compounds as mycotoxin biomarkers and give preliminary data from our work which aims at establishing an immunochemical strategy for biomonitoring of mycotoxins.

Keywords: mycotoxin, biomonitoring, blood, urine, immunoassay

A. Lindner (ed.) *Applied equine nutrition and training (ENUTRACO 2015)*
DOI 10.3920/978-90-8686-818-6_4, © Wageningen Academic Publishers 2015

Adverse effects of mycotoxins in horses

Mycotoxicoses in horses are a constant threat to equine health in many parts of the world. Obviously, the most important source of intake is mycotoxin ingestion via feedingstuffs and pasture. However, compared with livestock such as cattle, pigs and poultry, relatively few investigations have been done on equine species for most mycotoxins, with the big exception of the fumonisins. Nevertheless, the number of original studies on individual mycotoxins – in connection with equine intoxications – exceeds by far the framework of this presentation. Therefore, we refer to several excellent reviews on the current knowledge about the impact of mycotoxins on equine health (Caloni and Cortinovis, 2010, 2011; Hovermale and Craig, 2001; Marasas, 2001; Riet-Correa *et al.*, 2013). Riet-Correa *et al.* (2013) recently reviewed relevant literature on this topic, including mycotoxins produced on cereals after infection by fungi and by endophytic fungi in grasses, with special reference to South America. South America, as well as North America and South Africa, seem to be the regions with the highest number of reported mycotoxicoses in horses, mules and donkeys. In contrast, very few information on this topic is available from Europe. One factor explaining this situation may be sought in differences in feeding practices: in the Americas and South Africa, feeding of maize and maize by-products such as 'corn screenings', feeds that have a high risk of mycotoxin contamination, seems to be quite common (Ross *et al.*, 1991). On the other hand, awareness about equine mycotoxicoses may be less pronounced in horse owners and veterinarians in Europe, with the risk that some cases are overlooked.

The most notorious, and most specific, mycotoxicosis in equines is equine leukoencephalomalacia (ELEM), a disease caused by fumonisins, mycotoxins produced predominantly in maize by *Fusarium verticillioides*, *Fusarium proliferatum* and some other *Fusarium* species. The second important cause are ergot alkaloids and a variety of neurotoxic indole-diterpenoid toxins (produced by endophytic fungi such as *Neotyphodium* spp.) in grasses. Cases of aflatoxicosis in horses have been described (Caloni and Cortinovis, 2011), but seem to be less common, and aflatoxins may be comparatively less important in equines than in other species. The most abundant *Fusarium* toxins in many cereals in Europe and other parts of the world, deoxynivalenol (DON), zearalenone (ZEA), and T-2/HT-2-toxin, seem to have less pronounced toxicity towards horses than reported for other species (Caloni and Cortinovis, 2010).

Fusarium toxins

Fumonisins

Acute lethal intoxication of horses after feeding of maize contaminated with *F. verticillioides* (synonym *Fusarium moniliforme*), either through hepatotoxicity or through ELEM, has been known for long (Marasas, 2001). The clinical picture of ELEM is characterized by anorexia, dullness, drowsiness, hyperexcitability, blindness, ataxia and numerous other signs of neurological disorder (Riet-Correa *et al.*, 2013). The connection between *Fusarium*-infected maize and ELEM has been known at least since 1970, but only in 1988 fumonisin B_1 (FB_1) and its tumour-promoting activity was described, and FB_1 was only the first compound in a now long series of fumonisin mycotoxins (Marasas, 2001). Since then, liver damage and ELEM could be reproduced by feeding of FB_1 to horses, so that FB_1 is now considered as the causal agent of ELEM (Kellerman *et al.*, 1990; Marasas *et al.*, 1988). Equines seem to be the most sensitive species towards fumonisins, levels around 10 mg/kg or even lower in feed may induce ELEM. Maize, maize by-products or maize waste-products have been identified as the most important source of toxins (Marasas, 2001; Ross *et al.*, 1991). Case reports on ELEM originate predominantly from the Americas and South Africa (Table 1), while for Europe only a few reports have been published from Italy (Visconti *et al.*, 1995), Hungary (Fazekas and Bajmocy, 1996) and, most recently, from Serbia (Jovanović *et al.*, 2015). This is somehow surprising, because the number of horses in Germany is about 1 million (Liesener *et al.*, 2010); moreover, maize produced particularly in some parts of Europe may be heavily contaminated with fumonisins (Visconti *et al.*, 1995). The reason for this situation is not clear, but differences in feeding practices and in awareness of fumonisins may be contributing factors.

Trichothecenes and zearalenone

A few feeding studies have been performed to evaluate toxic effects in horses caused by the most common *Fusarium* toxins in cereals, namely trichothecenes such as DON and the oestrogenic ZEA.

M. Gross et al.

Table 1. Selected references describing confirmed cases of fumonisin-related equine leukoencephalomalacia in equines.

Country	Total number of animals/animals affected/lethal outcomes	Fumonisin levels in feed (mg/kg)	Year(s)[1]	Reference
USA	66/18/14	37-120 (FB_1); 2-23 (FB_2)	1989	Wilson et al., 1990
USA (45 cases)	>100/>100/>100	<1-126 (FB_1) (mostly >10)	1984-1990	Ross et al., 1991
Brazil (10 cases)	-/-/≥16	0.2-38.5 (FB_1); 0.1-12 (FB_2)	1985-1990	Sydenham et al., 1992
Italy	40/4/3	60 (FB_1); 15 (FB_2)	-	Visconti et al., 1995
Hungary	3/3/3	18.5 (FB_1)	1995	Fazekas and Bajmocy, 1996
Mexico	-/-/>100 (donkeys)	0.67-13.3 (FB_1)	-	Rosiles et al., 1998
Brazil	4/4/4	46-53 (FB_1)	1996	Mallmann et al., 1999
Brazil	28/6/6 (horses); 33/4/4 (mules)	6.6	2010	Dos Santos et al., 2013
Argentina	60/7/6	12.49 (FB_1); 5.25 (FB_2)	2007	Giannitti et al., 2011
Serbia	100/21/15	6-6.05 (FB_1); 1.68-2.4 (FB_2)	-	Jovanović et al., 2015

[1] Not indicated.

Unfortunately, these studies suffer from the fact that in nearly all cases naturally contaminated feed was used as the source of toxins. These materials usually contain several trichothecenes, ZEA and other *Fusarium* toxins simultaneously. Therefore, such studies reveal combined effects, coming from either the cytotoxic trichothecenes (feed refusal, reduced weight gain) or the hyperoestrogenic effects of ZEA (reproductive disorders) and possibly other toxins – the impact of individual toxins cannot be evaluated. The number of studies with horses is quite low, overviews have been compiled in some recent papers (Caloni and Cortinovis, 2010; Liesener, 2012; Songsermakul *et al.*, 2013). In general, horses seem to be less sensitive towards these toxins than other species, in particular less sensitive than pigs (D'Mello *et al.*, 1999).

Ergolines and endophyte toxins

In several regions of the world, intoxications with mycotoxins produced by endophytic fungi in pasture are a constant threat to equine health. These fungi can produce a range of toxic compounds which basically have insecticide or anti-herbivoric properties. Excellent reviews on this topic are available (Canty *et al.*, 2014; Plumlee and Galey, 1994; Riet-Correa *et al.*, 2013). While endophyte intoxications, such as ryegrass staggers, are very common in New Zealand and Australia (Imlach *et al.*, 2008) as well as in the Americas (Riet-Correa *et al.*, 2013), very few reports on this topic originate from Europe. However, endophyte toxins such as lolitrem and ergovaline have been found in pasture grasses in Germany (Oldenburg, 1997) and France (Repussard *et al.*, 2014). High levels of ergot alkaloids (exceeding 1 mg/kg) but not ergovaline have been reported for grasses (*Lolium perenne, Festuca arundinaceae*) from Germany (Riemel, 2012). The level of concern for lolitrem and ergovaline in grasses seems to be in a range of 2 mg/kg and 0.3-0.4 mg/kg, respectively (Hovermale and Craig, 2001). Feeding lolitrem at this level over several days reliably induced neurotoxic symptoms in horses (Johnstone *et al.*, 2012).

Ochratoxin A and aflatoxins

Little is known about possible toxic effects of ochratoxin A (OTA) in horses. Although it is a potent nephrotoxin in many species, and although it frequently occurs on cereals (Liesener *et al.*, 2010), we could not find a single report about ochratoxicosis in equines. Minervini *et al.* (2013) analysed blood serum from horses, including gravid mares, and found OTA in most animals,. However, levels were lower than those reported for most humans (Märtlbauer *et al.*, 2009). They could also confirm a placental transfer to the foals. Whether or not dietary OTA has any adverse effects in horses has yet to be confirmed.

Although cases of aflatoxicosis in horses have been described (Caloni and Cortinovis, 2011), the overall frequency seems to be quite low. Besides hepatotoxic and hepatocarcinogenic effects, it has been hypothesized that there could be a possible link between inhaled aflatoxins (from feed dust) and chronic obstructive pulmonary disease (COPD), however, an evidence has not been presented (Caloni and Cortinovis, 2011). With regard to mares as milk-producing animals for human consumption, the carry-over of aflatoxin metabolites, in particular aflatoxin M_1, into the milk would also be of interest, this aspect also has yet to be clarified.

Occurrence of mycotoxins in horse feed and environment

Horses may be exposed to mycotoxins originating from several sources. The question whether or not mycotoxins in dust or from other contaminated environmental materials may play a role in disease causation has not been clarified yet. In contrast, there is sufficient data showing that dietary exposure with mycotoxins can be the result of different sources.

First, the pasture may contain grasses such as *L. perenne* which contains mycotoxinogenic endophytic fungi. *Neotyphodium* species are known as important symbiontic fungi in *Poaceae*, in particular in the most robust grass species. Ergot alkaloids, namely ergovaline, as well as the neurotoxic indole-diterpenes lolitrem, paxilline (and others) may be present at levels that are sufficient to cause adverse effects (Riet-Correa *et al.*, 2013). Furthermore, if the grasses are allowed to grow during summer, ergot-producing *Claviceps* species may grow on nearly all *Poaceae* plants. This reflects the situation in the European Union, where farmers may receive subventions for not harvesting some of their pastures until late summer due to ecological and economic reasons. However, this also introduces another source of ergot alkaloids in grass and hay. The toxin levels in the ergot bodies growing on grasses may be quite high and easily result in levels exceeding 1 mg/g in the complete grass material (Riemel, 2012). If hay is produced from such grasses, the ergot alkaloid content might be reduced through UV light and storage, depending on the individual situation, but it is most likely that some of the toxic compounds remain in the hay.

Second, straw or other plant material used for bedding may also contain mycotoxins, *Fusarium* toxins in particular. Improper and wet storage of straw under cool weather conditions may favour growth of *Stachybotrys chartarum*, a producer of highly cytotoxic, macrocyclic trichothecenes such as satratoxin H. Large outbreaks of equine stachybotrycosis have been reported from Eastern Europe and from Hungary (Harrach *et al.*, 1987).

Third, horse stables may purchase oats, maize and other cereals from local farmers. These cereals are usually used 'as is', without mycotoxin analyses. We observed that in some cases such home-grown feedingstuffs may contain exceedingly high levels of *Fusarium* toxins, for example oats with T-2 and HT-2 toxin levels above 1 mg/kg.

Finally, commercial feedingstuffs for all levels of equine performance and age are available from a number of producers. It seems reasonable to assume that such feeds – or their ingredients – are at least randomly checked for those mycotoxins listed in European Union Commission Recommendations of 17 August 2006 (EC, 2006) and of 27 March 2013 (EC, 2013). For cereals and cereal products (with the exception of maize by-products), 'guidance values' are 8 mg/kg (DON), 2 mg/kg (ZEA), and 0.25 mg/kg (OTA). However, these are general values and have no direct reference to horse feed. The only specific guidance value for horses is available for fumonisins (5 mg/kg). For T-2 and HT-2 toxin in feeds, 'indicative levels' of 2 mg/kg in oat milling products (husks), 0.5 mg/kg in other cereals and 0.25 mg/kg in compound feeds have been recommended. Again, these indicative levels have no specific reference to horse feed.

Some years ago, Liesener *et al.* (2010) performed a systematic monitoring study on various types of commercially available horse feeds (muesli, mash, pellets, plain cereals) in Germany. In their study, the median values for all types of feedingstuffs were far below the guidance values; even the maximum values found in some samples (mostly plain cereals) were well below the guidance values and indicative values (Figure 1). It has to be emphasized that – except for the fumonisins – recommendations on maximum mycotoxin levels in horse feed are more or less educated guesses, because of the scarcity of toxicological data.

One major finding of Liesener *et al.* (2010) was the presence of ergot alkaloids at low levels in the majority of samples, the maximum level found in one barley sample (1.2 mg/kg) was quite high. Another remarkable aspect was that the highest concentrations of DON, ZEA and fumonisins were all found in plain maize feed. In composed feeds, the concentrations of all mycotoxins did not correlate well with any cereal ingredient. From our and literature data, it seems to

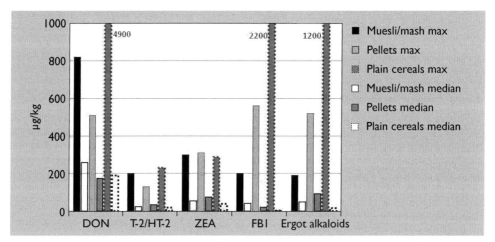

Figure 1. Mycotoxins in commercial horse feeds in Germany (64 different batches from different producers; data taken from Liesener et al., 2010). Even the maximum values are lower than the guidance values given in European Union Commission Recommendations (EC, 2006 and 2013).

be advisable to avoid maize as much as possible in horse feeding, in particular maize by-products such as 'corn screenings' or 'grain dust'.

If an analysis of the mycotoxin risk for a given herd is needed, or if mycotoxins are suspected as the cause of disease in horses, reliance on mycotoxin feed analyses has several disadvantages:

- The feed sample under analysis may not be representative for the feed ingested, because of heterogeneous distribution of toxins. Such heterogeneity possibly also applies to endophyte-infected pastures.
- The feed sample under analysis may not even be related to the true source of feed, because a highly toxic batch may have been replaced with a less toxic one between intoxication and sampling. Furthermore, if both home-grown and commercial feeds are used, it will be most likely the commercial feed and not the home-grown feed which will be sent for mycotoxin analysis.
- It is possible that none of the most obvious feedingstuffs but something else (bedding, grain or straw dust, fruits, carrots) is the true source of mycotoxins.

As an alternative to feed analysis, the overall level of exposure to mycotoxins by a certain horse or a herd of horses could be controlled, if (1) suitable biomarkers can be identified, and (2) a cost-efficient method of analysis is available. The best example for successful mycotoxin biomonitoring is OTA in blood serum of humans, which can give information about the dietary intake of this toxin (Märtlbauer *et al.*, 2009). Moreover, multi-mycotoxin exposure through all sources of ingestion can be performed, which is important considering the possible synergistic or additive effects of mycotoxins. Such studies have recently been performed for urine from humans (Gerding *et al.*, 2014; Solfrizzo *et al.*, 2014).

Immunochemical biomonitoring of mycotoxins

Few studies on mycotoxin levels in biological material from horses have been published so far. OTA, which strongly binds to serum albumin in many mammalian species, has been found at low levels of around 0.1 ng/ml in 83% of blood serum samples of horses (Minervini *et al.*, 2013). These levels are somewhat lower than in humans, in which OTA levels in blood samples are an excellent biomarker of exposure (Märtlbauer *et al.*, 2009).

Exposure of horses towards aflatoxin might frequently occur on a worldwide basis; some cases of aflatoxicosis in horses have been described (Caloni and Cortinovis, 2011) At least in middle Europe heavily aflatoxin-contaminated feed material is probably of rare occurrence. Data on blood and urine levels as biomarkers for aflatoxins in horses could not be found, furthermore, it is likely that aflatoxin M_1 rather than aflatoxin B_1 would be present.

In 1992, an altered ratio between sphingosin/sphinganine and complex sphingolipids has been observed in ponies given feed containing fumonisins, because these toxins disrupt sphingolipid metabolism (Wang *et al.*, 1992). An increased ratio of sphingosin to sphinganine and other shifts in sphingosin metabolism have been suggested as early biomarkers of fumonisin exposure (Shephard *et al.*, 2007). A drawback of these approaches is the high physiological variability of sphingolipid levels between individuals, as well as within one individual over time, making the interpretation of data difficult. Fumonisin is poorly absorbed and excreted mostly via the faeces. Levels in blood serum and urine seem to be relatively low. Fumonisin analysis in serum and urine has therefore been considered as less useful. However, provided that an analytical method for fumonisins in urine is sensitive enough, this approach could still be useful to detect acute and high fumonisin exposure (Van der Westhuizen *et al.*, 2011).

For the metabolism of ZEA in the horse, Songsermsakul *et al.* (2013) detected β-zearalenol (β-ZOL) in plasma at high levels, while β-ZOL and α-ZOL were the major metabolites in urine, nearly all as glucuronides. For DON and other trichothecenes, the parent compounds, their deepoxy metabolites, and glucuronides/sulfonates thereof may be found in serum and urine (Gerding *et al.*, 2014). For ergot alkaloids, no data could be found concerning biomarkers in blood serum or urine of horses.

Recent approaches towards detection of mycotoxin biomarkers in urine or serum use LC-MS/MS methods (Gerding *et al.*, 2014); the increased sensitivity of this equipment often allows dilute-and-shoot approach, avoiding time-consuming sample preparation. However, LC-MS/MS methods are still very costly, multiple analyses are time-consuming, and testing outside specialized laboratories is not possible. In the last decades, immunochemical methods of detection for mycotoxins such as enzyme immunoassays (EIA) have been developed for most major mycotoxins. These methods enable low-cost analysis of single or multiple samples at a sensitive level of detection. A possible disadvantage is a varying and sometimes unpredictable cross-reactivity with metabolites, making quantitative analyses questionable when several compounds are present at the same time. However, if the ratio of metabolites in a biological sample is relatively stable, the numerical data obtained from the EIA standard curve still give a good indicator value, thus allowing a discrimination between high and low exposure levels. At the moment, it is quite unclear for which mycotoxins EIA detection in serum and urine would be useful. Furthermore, neither 'normal' or 'harmless' values nor levels of concern for mycotoxins in these biological matrices have been established yet.

We therefore started a screening study, using a set of sensitive EIA methods and a larger number of blood serum and urine samples of sport horses, of which we assume that the vast majority will not suffer from elevated levels of mycotoxins. This should provide a first idea about the span of a normal range of mycotoxin data and give a first set of normal blood and urine of horses in Germany.

The sample material was provided by the Deutsche Sporthochschule Köln (German Sport University Cologne, Institute for Biochemistry), which is responsible for doping control of sport horses. In the years 2013/2014, a total of 100 blood samples and 200 urine samples were obtained for analysis. The parameters analysed so far are DON, ZEA, ergonovine, fumonisin (FB_1) and OTA. All mycotoxins were analysed by enzyme immunoassays (EIA). For analysis of DON and ZEA, samples were pretreated with glucuronidase/sulfatase (100 U/ml, 2 h, 37 °C) before extract preparation. Details on these EIAs have been given by Liesener *et al.* (2010). The detection limit for the parent toxin in urine and serum was nearly identical for DON and ZEA, whereas for ergonovine and OTA a tenfold more sensitive detection was achieved in blood serum (Table 2).

Table 2. Preliminary data of the immunochemical screening study on mycotoxins in samples of blood serum (n=100) and urine (n=200) of sport horses from Germany.

Parameter	Result enzyme immunoassays test system for				
	Deoxynivalenol	Ergonovine	Fumonisin B_1	Ochratoxin A	Zearalenone
Detection limit in blood, ng/ml	12	0.01	-[a]	0.05	1.0
Detection limit in urine, ng/ml	12	0.16	0.5	0.5	1.0
Mean recovery from blood and urine, %	86	68	110	72	82
Blood serum: mean ± SD levels of positive samples (maximum value), ng/ml	16.6[b]	0.019±0.007 (0.032)	-	0.10±0.055 (0.28)	1.41±0.60 (2.70)
Urine: mean ± SD levels of positive samples (maximum value), ng/ml	82.4±55.8 (487)	0.55±0.23 (39.8)	0.55±0.27 (1.0)	0.16±0.08 (2.80)	10.5±7.34 (20.3)

[a] Not determined.

[b] One positive sample only.

Table 2 also gives an overview about the results obtained so far. Figure 2 illustrates the frequency of positive results in each test system for blood and urine. Blood serum was frequently positive only for OTA and ergonovine, DON and ZEA were positive in a few samples only, fumonisins have not yet been analysed. Urine samples were for all toxins more frequently positive (70-95%), even the FB_1-EIA yielded 10% positive results. The mean levels in urine for all toxins were well above the EIA detection limits. The results indicate that urine is probably a better sample matrix to study exposure of horses to the five mycotoxins than blood serum. Since most EIAs – except the OTA-EIA – cross-react with metabolites, the data as shown in Table 2 have to be regarded as preliminary indicator values, until the metabolite profile is more clearly understood in horses.

In agreement with results from an earlier study on mycotoxins in horse feed, the data suggest that horses are continuously exposed to multiple mycotoxins (Liesener *et al.*, 2010). However, further studies are necessary to correlate mycotoxin levels in urine with feed intake data. Further work will include analyses of more toxins for which EIA tests are available, including aflatoxins, sterigmatocystin, paxilline and alternariol.

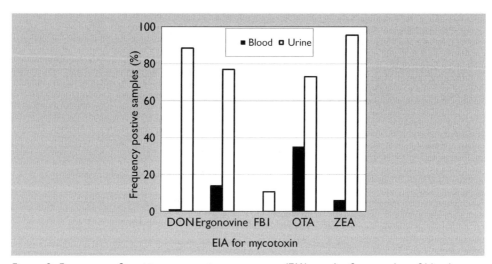

Figure 2. Frequency of positive enzyme immunoassays (EIA) results for samples of blood serum (n=100) and urine (n=200) of horses from Germany. Data for blood serum in the FB_1-EIA have not yet been obtained.

Conclusions

Fumonisins in maize as well as ergot alkaloids and indole-diterpenes in endophyte-infected grasses are presumably the most important mycotoxins in aspects of equine health. While fumonisin intake can be reduced by avoiding maize, contaminated pasture is a problem which is less easy to solve. Because the overall exposure of horses to mycotoxins is difficult to assess by feed analysis, biomonitoring of biological material (blood serum, urine) offers an interesting alternative here. However, at the moment basic data that would enable a practical search strategy and a sound interpretation are lacking. Our first results in an approach to establish an immunochemical biomonitoring system for mycotoxin exposure of horses, using a set of mycotoxin EIAs, indicate that equine urine could be a useful matrix to assess overall multi-mycotoxin exposure.

Acknowledgments

We thank the Verein zur Förderung der Forschung im Pferdesport (FFP) e.V. for the financial support.

References

Caloni, F. and Cortinovis, C., 2010. Effects of fusariotoxins in the equine species. Veterinary Journal 186: 157-161.

Caloni, F. and Cortinovis, C., 2011. Toxicological effects of aflatoxins in horses. Veterinary Journal 188: 270-273.

Canty, M.J., Fogarty, U., Sheridan, M.K., Ensley, S.M., Schrunk, D.E. and More, S.J., 2014. Ergot alkaloid intoxication in perennial rye grass (*Lolium perenne*): an emerging animal health concern in Ireland? Irish Veterinary Journal 67: 1-7.

D´Mello, J.P.F., Placinta, C.M. and Macdonald, A.M.C., 1999. *Fusarium* mycotoxins: a review of global implications for animal health, welfare and productivity. Animal Feed Science and Technology 80: 183-205.

Dos Santos, C.E.P., Souto, F.S.M., Santurio, J.M. and Marques, L.C., 2013. Leucoencefalomalácia em equídeos da região leste de mato grosso. Acta Scientiae Veterinariae 41: 1-6.

European Commission (EC), 2006. Commission Recommendation of 17 August 2006 on the presence of deoxynivalenol, zearalenone, ochratoxin A, T-2 and HT-2 and fumonisins in products intended for animal feeding (2006/576/EC). Official Journal of the European Union L 229: 7-9.

European Commission (EC), 2013. Commission Recommendation of 27 March 2013 on the presence of T-2 and HT-2 toxin in cereals and cereal products (2013/165/EU). Official Journal of the European Union L 91: 12-15.

Fazekas, B. and Bajmocy, G., 1996. Occurrence of the equine leukoencephalomalacia (ELEM) caused by fumonisin-B-1 mycotoxin in Hungary. Magyar Allatorvosok Lapja 51: 484-487.

Gerding, J., Cramer, B. and Humpf, H.U., 2014. Determination of mycotoxin exposure in Germany using an LC-MS/MS multibiomarker approach. Molecular Nutrition and Food Research 58: 2358-2368.

Giannitti, F., Sain Diab, S., Pacin, A.M., Barrandeguy, M., Larrere, C., Ortega, J. and Uzal, F.A., 2011. Equine leukoencephalomalacia (ELEM) due to fumonisins B_1 and B_2 in Argentina. Pesquisa Veterinária Brasileira 31: 407-412.

Harrach, B., Bata, A., Sandor, G. and Vanyi, A., 1987. Isolation of macrocyclic and non-macrocyclic trichothecenes (*Stachybotrys* and *Fusarium* toxins) from the environment of 200 sport horses. Mycotoxin Research 3: 65-68.

Hovermale, J.T. and Craig, M., 2001. Correlation of ergovaline and lolitrem B levels in endophyte-infected perennial ryegrass (*Lolium perenne*). Journal of Veterinary Diagnostic Investigation 13: 323-327.

Imlach, W.L., Finch, S.C., Dunlop, J., Meredith, A.L., Aldrich, R.W. and Dalziel, J.E., 2008. The molecular mechanism of 'ryegrass staggers,' a neurological disorder of K^+ channels. Journal of Pharmacology and Experimental Therapeutics 327: 657-664.

Johnstone, L.K., Mayhew, I.G. and Fletcher, L.R., 2012. Clinical expression of lolitrem B (perennial ryegrass) intoxication in horses. Equine Veterinary Journal 44: 304-309.

Jovanović, M., Trailović, D., Kukolj, V., Marinković, D., Nedeljković-Trailović, J., Jakovac Strajn, B. and Milićević, D., 2015. An outbreak of fumonisin toxicosis in horses in Serbia. World Mycotoxin Journal 8: 387-391.

Kellerman, T.S., Marasas, W.F.O., Thiel, P.G., Gelderblom, W.C.A., Cawood, M. and Coetzer, J.A.W., 1990. Leukoencephalomalacia in two horses induced by oral dosing of fumonisin B_1. Onderstepoort Journal of Veterinary Research 57: 269-275.

Liesener, K., Curtui, V., Dietrich, R., Märtlbauer, E. and Usleber, E., 2010. Mycotoxins in horse feed. Mycotoxin Research 26: 23-30.

Liesener, K., 2012. Untersuchung zum Nachweis und zum Vorkommen von Mykotoxinen in Futtermitteln für Pferde. Thesis, Veterinary Faculty, University of Giessen, Germany.

Märtlbauer, E., Usleber, E., Dietrich, R. and Schneider, E., 2009. Ochratoxin A in human blood serum – retrospective long-term data. Mycotoxin Research 25: 175-186.

Mallmann, C.A., Santurio, J.M. and Dilkin, P., 1999. Equine leukoencephalomalacia associated with ingestion of corn contaminated with fumonisin B_1. Revista de Microbiologia 30: 249-252.

Marasas, W.F.O., Kellerman, T.S., Gelderblom, W.C.A., Coetzer, J.A.W., Thiel, P.G. and Van der Lugt, J.J., 1988. Leukoencephalomalacia in a horse induced by fumonisin B_1 isolated from *Fusarium moniliforme*. Onderstepoort Journal of Veterinary Research 55: 197-203.

Marasas, W.F.O., 2001. Discovery and occurrence of the fumonisins: a historical perspective. Environmental Health Perspectives 109: 239-243.

Minervini, F., Giannoccaro A., Nicassio, M., Panzarini, G. and Lacalandra, G.M., 2013. First evidence of placental transfer of ochratoxin A in horses. Toxins 5: 84-92.

Oldenburg, E., 1997. Endophytic fungi and alkaloid production in perennial ryegrass in Germany. Grass and Forage Science 52: 425-431.

Plumlee, K.H. and Galey, F.D., 1994. Neurotoxic mycotoxins: a review of fungal toxins that cause neurological disease in large animals. Journal of Veterinary Internal Medicine 8: 49-54.

Repussard, C., Zbib, N., Tardieu, D. and Guerre, P., 2014. Ergovaline and lolitrem B concentrations in perennial ryegrass in field culture in southern France: distribution in the plant and impact of climatic factors. Journal of Agricultural and Food Chemistry 62: 12707-12712.

Riemel, J., 2012. Untersuchungen zum Nachweis und zum Vorkommen von Ergotalkaloiden in Futtergräsern. Thesis, Veterinary Faculty, University of Giessen, Germany.

Riet-Correa, F., Rivero, R., Odriozola, E., De Lourdes Adrien, M., Medeiros, R.M.T. and Schild, A.L., 2013. Mycotoxicoses of ruminants and horses. Journal of Veterinary Diagnostic Investigation 25: 692-708.

Rosiles, M.R., Bautista, J., Fuentes, V.O. and Ross, F., 1998. An outbreak of equine leukoencephalomalacia at Oaxaca, Mexico, associated with fumonisin B_1. Journal of Veterinary Medicine Series A 45: 299-302.

Ross, P.F., Rice, L.G., Reagor, J.C., Osweiler, G.D., Wilson, T.M., Nelson, H.A., Owens, D.L., Plattner, R.D., Harlin, K.A., Richard, J.L., Colvin, B.M. and Banton, M.I., 1991. Fumonisin B_1 concentrations in feeds from 45 confirmed equine leukoencephalomalacia cases. Journal of Veterinary Diagnostic Investigation 3: 238-241.

Shepard, G.S., Van der Westhuizen, L. and Sewram A., 2007: Biomoarkers of exposure to fumonisin mycotoxins. A review. Food Additives and Contaminants 24: 1196-1201.

Solfrizzo, M., Gambacorta, L. and Visconti, A., 2014. Assessment of multi-mycotoxin exposure in southern Italy by urinary multi-biomarker determination. Toxins 6: 523-538.

Songsermsakul, P., Böhm, J., Aurich, C., Zentek, J. and Razzazi-Fazeli, E., 2013. The levels of zearalenone and its metabolites in plasma, urine and faeces of horses fed with naturally, *Fusarium* toxin-contaminated oats. Journal of Animal Physiology and Animal Nutrition 97: 155-161.

Sydenham, E.W., Marasas, W.F.O., Shepard, G.S., Thiel, P.G. and Hirooka, E.Y., 1992. Fumonisin concentrations in Brazilian feeds associated with field outbreaks of confirmed and suspected animal mycotoxicoses. Journal of Agricultural and Food Chemistry 40: 994-997.

Van der Westhuizen, L., Shephard, G.S., Burger, H.M., Rheeder, J.P, Gelderblom, W.C.A., Wild, C.P., and Gong, Y.Y., 2011. Fumonisin B_1 as a urinary biomarker of exposure in a maize intervention study among South African subsistence farmers. Cancer Epidemiology, Biomarkers and Prevention 20: 483-489.

Visconti, A., Boenke, A., Doko, M.B., Solfrizzo, M. and Pascale, M., 1995. Occurrence of fumonisins in Europe and the BCR-measurements and testing projects. Natural Toxins 3: 269-274.

Wang, E., Ross, P.F., Wilson, T.M., Riley, R.T. and Merrill, A.H., 1992. Increases in serum sphingosine and sphinganine and decreases in complex sphingolipids in ponies given feed containing fumonisins, mycotoxins produced by *Fusarium moniliforme*. Journal of Nutrition 122: 1706-1716.

Wilson, T.M., Ross, P.F., Rice, L.G., Osweiler, G.D., Nelson, H.A., Owens, D.L., Plattner, R.D., Reggiardo, C., Noon, T.H. and Pickrell, J.W., 1990. Fumonisin B_1 levels associated with an epizootic of equine leukoencephalomalacia. Journal of Veterinary Diagnostic Investigation 2: 213-216.

5. The whole horse approach to equine physical rehabilitation: the biomechanical view

S.J. Schils[1]* and D. Isbell[2]
[1]EquiNew, 8139 900th Street, River Falls, WI 54022, USA; [2]P.O. Box 671, Livermore, CA 94551, USA; sbschils@equinew.com

Abstract

When the biomechanics of movement of the whole horse is evaluated during rehabilitation, the chance of a successful outcome increases. Faulty movement can be caused by conformation, injury and/or imbalanced work. Faulty movement induces pain and pain induces faulty movement. These related issues result in weakness of the tissues associated with the pain and incorrect movement. As weakness is the symptom of the inciting problem, strengthening alone only treats the symptom. Locating and treating the cause, especially the mechanical cause of pain, is an important part of a rehabilitation protocol. Strengthening of muscles, tendons and ligaments is a common goal of a rehabilitation program. However, too much strength can be as detrimental to healing and injury prevention as too little strength, and can disrupt the biomechanical balance of the body. Flexibility is necessary to keep joint movement smooth and to retain range of motion. However, hypermobility can be a major cause of injury and is a typical outcome when hypomobility has produced limited range of motion in one area of the body. The excessive movement of hypermobility can cause degenerative joint disease leading to compensatory movement and further pain. Diagnostic ultrasound is a quick, safe, economical and effective means of diagnosing a variety of issues in equine medicine and is the optimal method for monitoring the progression of healing in these injuries. Physical rehabilitation takes time, but simply allowing more time for the rehabilitation process is not the answer.

Keywords: flexibility, muscle, joint, strength, tendon, ultrasound

A. Lindner (ed.) *Applied equine nutrition and training (ENUTRACO 2015)*
DOI 10.3920/978-90-8686-818-6_5, © Wageningen Academic Publishers 2015

Introduction

The science of physical rehabilitation takes the basis of knowledge from biomechanics, kinesiology and anatomy, and adds to that a practical clinical application. Physical rehabilitation is not just rest with a gradual increase in work. Rather, the science of rehabilitation takes into account information that we have learned about the mechanics of movement, how tissues heal, and in what environment they heal the best. The goal of a quality rehabilitation protocol is to apply information from a variety of scientific fields to offer the patient the best opportunity to obtain the highest quality of healing.

Biomechanics is defined as the mechanics of a biological system, using the basis of physics to understand movement. Biomechanics can be helpful in breaking down the complex movement of the body into singular concepts that are more easily evaluated. Physical rehabilitation for the equine athlete is an important means of retaining the value of the horse as well as improving the quality of the horse's life. The purpose of this paper is to look at how the concepts of biomechanics can help us better understand the theories of equine rehabilitation.

What is the whole horse approach to rehabilitation?

Looking at the entire horse to evaluate a physical rehabilitation plan is a realistic goal. However, we tend to concentrate on the areas of the horse that we are the most comfortable in evaluating. For example, a kinesiologist will focus on the muscular components that are causing pain and may overlook the heel bruise that is the primary cause of the lameness. Or the clinical veterinarian will determine that the cause of lameness is adhesions of the deep digital tendon sheath and miss the muscular shoulder asymmetry producing incorrect loading of the limb. Combining the skills of several experts is an obvious advantage when developing a rehabilitation plan.

Diagnostic ultrasound monitoring of soft tissue injuries, avulsion fractures and bone surface remodelling can enable a more accurate assessment of the injury than can be done with less objective means, such as heat, swelling or pain. Using ultrasound, one can evaluate the stage of healing and the level of motion and load that the tissue can withstand without reinjury. Serial ultrasound imaging throughout the rehabilitation period can determine if the work is excessive and may cause reinjury, or if the work is correct and the tissues are healing appropriately (Gillis, 1997). Small changes in ultrasonographic parameters of size, echogenicity, and fibre pattern are associated with a relatively large change in anatomical parameters (Gillis, 2004).

What is the biomechanical focus of the whole horse approach to rehabilitation?

The whole horse body mechanics should always be evaluated weather the diagnosis is overriding dorsal spinal processes or a distal limb pathology. For example, if the diagnosis is an epaxial muscle tear, the loading of the limbs and the swing and stance pattern of the stride should also be thoroughly examined. Even during the hand walking stage of rehabilitation, the horse should be carefully monitored to reduce abnormal limb loading and swing patterns. Conversely, if the diagnosis is a distal limb problem, the epaxial muscles should be evaluated for symmetry, hypertension and atrophy of the musculoskeletal system.

Muscle memory patterns have been shown to be an adaptation of the neuromuscular system (Chapman *et al.*, 2007; Wakeling and Horn, 2009). Therefore, the muscle pattern recognition can be very strong, especially when the pattern has been established at an early age, and changing movement patterns takes time and repetition (Halsband and Lange, 2006). Rehabilitation programs that occur over an extended period of time and emphasize quality movement will have a better chance of success.

Ultrasound can identify the size, shape, echogenicity (grey scale that enables the detection of oedema, normal tissue, and scar tissue), bone reaction at soft tissue attachments, joint and bursa effusion, synovial proliferation and capsule thickness. Fibre pattern, showing the parallel alignment of tendon and ligament fibres, is an indication of tissue strength (Gigante *et al.*, 2009) and can be monitored via ultrasound throughout the rehabilitation period. Serial imaging facilitates assessment of tissue structure to determine if the rehabilitation work is overloading the injured tissues or is enabling healing for return to function.

Pain

When body movement is not ideal, limitations in movement occur and the body will start to change the biomechanically correct manner in which it functions, resulting in pain and breakdown of the musculoskeletal system (Van Dillen *et al.*, 2007). Late-stage structural faults of the body typically begin as alignment faults and pain does not usually occur until the alignment fault becomes severe (Spitznagel and Ivens, 2011).

Unfortunately, just removing the pain will not automatically solve the problem if the incorrect mechanics are not addressed. Pain may cause the movement of the horse to change as a consequence of injury (Sterling *et al.*, 2001), or incorrect biomechanical movement may result in pain (Sahrmann, 2002). In addition, if the pain is due to compensatory issues, dealing with only the site of the initial injury will not heal the horse. If the pain is removed, the horse can be returned to work, and may do so happily. However, once the pain is removed, continuing to work the horse without correcting the cause of the pain may make future problems worse. It is important to correct the painful movement pattern rather than just treating the painful tissues. For example, if a horse with cervical joint disease is treated with injections and is then put back to full work, the treatment can actually cause a progression of the disease. Due to the joint disease, the muscles supporting the cervical spine are atrophied and/or in hypertension. Asking the horse to return to work after removing the joint pain without providing the correct supportive musculature, worsens the degenerative joint disease. This is due to the fact that the abnormal movement pattern has not been corrected. Therefore, the next injection doesn't work as well or last as long and the degenerative cycle continues until the horse must be retired. If before and after the horse is injected there is a period of careful muscle strengthening, while maintaining alignment, then the horse can return to work without the joint instability that is detrimental to healing. Continuing specific exercises to maintain appropriate muscle function for joint stability and alignment enables the horse to remain in work without, or with minimal, progression in joint degeneration.

Stance-phase and swing-phase of the limb

Stance-phase lameness and swing-phase lameness differentiation is another means of pinpointing the source of the lameness. In stance-phase lameness, the discomfort occurs during weight bearing, and in swing-phase lameness, the discomfort occurs during the unweighted movement of the limb. In general, swing-phase lameness has a distinct muscular dysfunction as the cause (Piazza and Delp, 1996). Swing phase of the stride has not been studied extensively due to the early impression that this element of the stride was simply a pendulum effect.

The distinction between swing-phase lameness and stance-phase lameness has led to improved diagnostic and treatment regimes in rehabilitation (Lam *et al.*, 2008). A recent study in humans has shown that the hamstrings of sprinters are most susceptible to injury during the late swing phase of the stride (Chumanov *et al.*, 2012). In addition, correction of swing-phase pathology will typically improve the stance phase of the limb.

In biomechanics, the first evaluation of incorrect movement is to examine the way the limb contacts the ground in the stance phase. The structure of the foot, the shoe and the surfaces that the foot is in contact with during stance, are of primary concern. Secondly, the evaluation moves to the swing phase where observation is focused on the movement proximal to the core to determine any defects. Third, evaluations of the swing phase are made in succession moving incrementally distal. Fourth, evaluation of the stance phase continues with observations being made proximal to distal to identify problems. This rehabilitation structure is based on the biomechanical principle that distal structures are most influenced by the type of rotation closest to the centre of the structure. Therefore, during rehabilitation influencing the centre of rotation influences the distal limb.

Balancing muscle movement

Diagnosis of the specific problem, or problems, is essential, however during the rehabilitation plan, focus is not just placed on the site of the injury. Agonistic and antagonist muscles are of equal importance when trying to improve the faulty movement pattern that is typically present when injury occurs (Scholtes *et al.*, 2010). At times, working the antagonist muscle relative to the injured muscle is more advantageous than working specifically on the site of injury. For example, if the horse has experienced a muscle tear during contraction of the biceps the focus can be on strengthening the triceps to elongate the biceps during healing to help reduce scar tissue and adhesions.

Strength versus flexibility

Strengthening during rehabilitation is emphasized in most protocols, but in many situations over strengthening of one area is the reason the injury occurred initially. The over strengthened area results in limited mobility in that region which leads to hypermobility in a related region of the body to compensate for this lack of movement (Lotz and Ulrich, 2006). To heal the injury it is sometimes necessary to obtain more flexibility at the primary injury site, while strengthening occurs at an associated area.

To gain joint stability, the balance of flexibility and strength should be emphasized. The major factor in cartilage degeneration appears to be stresses on the synovium due to joint instability rather than inflammation (Lukoschek *et al.*, 1986). Stabilization of the joint will not occur with rest, rather the opposite will be true (Spitznagle and Ivens, 2011). In humans, if braces are used early in the stabilisation process to protect the site of injury these braces should allow movement of the joint. However, the braces must allow biomechanically correct movement and not just support the incorrect movement patterns that caused the injury in the first place.

Symmetry of movement

One major cause of breakdown is not the number of repetitions of a movement pattern, but rather the number of biomechanically incorrect movements. Asymmetry of movement causes significant biomechanical alignment problems in the body leading to injury (Guilak *et al.*, 2004). Symmetry of motion is the foundation of quality movement, and quality movement is a very important element of long-term pain-free movement (Gombatto *et al.*, 2008). Symmetry must be evaluated based on the specific movement, but sagittal plane symmetry is a quality to strive for.

Rotation

Torque is sometimes referred to as rotation, but it is actually the force that causes the movement which then results in biomechanically correct or pathological rotation. Pathological rotation quickly deteriorates joints and although it is not always associated with asymmetrical movement, the two issues are distinctly related (Lukoschek *et al.*, 1986). For example, in humans, pathological rotation of the thorax is a major factor in patients with neck pain (Sahrmann and Bloom, 2011). In the horse, observation of the rotation in the pelvis can be an important indicator of the pressures placed on the stifle and hock, and vice versa.

Hypermobility and hypomobility

Many times when a horse is palpated, the site of minimal movement is thought to be the main problem area. However, as we look at new research, we see that hypermobility can be an important forbearer of injury (Sahrmann and Bloom, 2011). As hypermobility continues, the joint breaks down and the muscles begin to spasm due to overwork, leading to further complications. The end result is hypomobility where the degenerative process has resulted in the loss of cartilage and exostosis (Adams and Dolan, 1995). An initial reduction in hypermobility, to improve stability, can be necessary before the hypomobility can be addressed. This theory is now widely accepted in human rehabilitation, however, when it was first introduced the concept was dismissed (Sahrmann and Bloom, 2011).

Ground reaction force

Ground reaction force is a major concern during rehabilitation and due to the pressures exerted to the repairing structures, it should be. However, research has shown that the body can handle higher concussionary forces than previously thought, as long as the force is applied in a biomechanically correct manner (Rupp *et al.*, 2010). If forces are increased gradually, and are within acceptable ranges, adaption can occur which can increase tendon, muscle and bone strength (Woo *et al.*, 1987).

The horse's suspensory ligament can sustain a pound force of about 3,500 when landing over a 4-foot jump (Meershoek *et al.*, 2010). Studies have shown that at high speeds of the gallop the superficial flexor tendons have a small margin of biomechanical safety between tolerance and breakdown (Dowling and Dart, 2005), while the extensor tendons have a larger margin of safety (Batson *et al.*, 2003). Problems arise when pathological rotational forces, due to poor alignment, are also present during concussion. Musculoskeletal tissues are not designed to accept the asymmetrical forces, and breakdown quickly occurs.

The type of surface used in a rehabilitation program is important when evaluating how to obtain the desired ground reaction forces. In human studies, the firm surface of clay produced fewer injuries, compared to grass and asphalt, when injuries were evaluated in tennis players (Bastholt, 2000). In addition, studies in horses have shown that a soft surface, which deforms considerably, can increase physical demands of work and induce an earlier onset of fatigue (Sloet van Oldruitenborgh-Oosterbaan *et al.*, 1991).

Proprioception

Proprioception is the neuromuscular response that causes muscles to react appropriately without conscious effort. Proprioception is one of the first reactions of the body to diminish with immobilization (Hewett *et al.*, 2002). With proprioception retraining after injury, the horse has a reduced chance of reinjury when the footing becomes uneven, or they lose their balance, especially at speed. Challenging the balance of the horse by reasonably working the horse in uneven footing, in lateral exercises, over a variety of surfaces and up and down hills, as a few examples, will assist in improving the horse's proprioception during rehabilitation.

Conclusions

Shirley Sahrmann, a leader in physical rehabilitation theory and techniques for people, has summarised how motor control is related to movement asymmetries, which is related to pain syndromes. She states that 'the critical factor is not what you do as much as how you do it' (Sahrmann and Bloom, 2011).

When the biomechanics of movement of the whole horse is evaluated during rehabilitation, the chance of a successful outcome increases. For example, if the distinct asymmetry in the scapula is not addressed, the prognosis of the front suspensory tear will be guarded. This is due to the fact that the pathological loading of the limb caused by the asymmetrical body biomechanics has not been corrected.

Faulty movement can be caused by conformation, injury and/or imbalanced work. Faulty movement induces pain and pain induces faulty movement. These related issues result in weakness of the tissues associated with the pain and incorrect movement. As weakness is the symptom of the inciting problem, strengthening alone only treats the symptom. Locating and treating the cause, especially the mechanical cause of pain, is an important part of a rehabilitation protocol.

The causes of swing- and stance-phase lameness are distinctly different when viewed biomechanically. Swing-phase lameness is the most easily overlooked and typically has a muscular component, which can be the primary or secondary cause of movement dysfunction. If swing-phase corrections are made, a difference in loading will also be seen. Therefore, if only stance phase corrections are made, the cause of the lameness may not be completely addressed.

Asymmetrical movement and pathological rotations are two of the primary reasons for injury. Strengthening of muscles, tendons and ligaments is a common goal of a rehabilitation program. However, too much strength can be as detrimental to healing and injury prevention as too little strength, and can disrupt the biomechanical balance of the body. When strengthening does not improve the symmetry of the body, the effect of the strengthening exercises can result in uneven loading and stress on the musculoskeletal system.

Flexibility is necessary to keep joint movement smooth and to retain range of motion. However, hypermobility can be a major cause of injury. Hypermobility is a typical outcome when hypomobility has produced a limited range of motion in one area of the body. To compensate for this inhibition of joint movement, the associated joints have excessive movement. The excessive movement causes degenerative joint disease leading to compensatory movement and further pain. Ground reaction forces are important issues to consider, however studies have shown that the body can handle higher concussionary forces than previously thought. Both hard and soft surfaces are responsible for injuries although the types of injuries vary based on the surface. For soft tissue injuries, firm surfaces are being viewed as producing fewer injuries when compared to softer or harder surfaces.

Diagnostic ultrasound is a quick, safe, economical and effective means of diagnosing a variety of issues in equine medicine. The majority of equine injuries include soft tissue damage and ultrasound is the optimal method for diagnosing and monitoring the progression of healing in these injuries. Ultrasound can identify many of the upper body issues, such as spinal and muscle problems that cannot be imaged with any other modality due to the size of the horse. Ultrasound is effective at identifying subtle bone surface changes such as osteophytes, enthesiopathies, avulsion fractures, periosteal reaction, callous formation, and stress fractures. In addition, through sequential ultrasounds structural changes can be monitored throughout the healing process.

Physical rehabilitation takes time, but simply allowing more time for the rehabilitation process is not the answer. The science of physical rehabilitation is complex and constantly evolving and requires knowledgeable evaluation and application. Many caregivers through trial and error have learned valuable techniques and protocols that should be evaluated as we bring together clinical and research concepts.

References

Adams, M.A. and Dolan P., 1995. Recent advances in lumbar spinal mechanics and their clinical significance. Clinical Biomechanics 10: 3-1.

Batson, E.L., Paramour, R.J., Smith, T.J., Birch, H.L., Patterson-Kane, J.C. and Goodship, A.E., 2003. Are the material properties and matrix composition of equine flexor and extensor tendons determined by their functions? Equine Veterinary Journal 35: 314-318.

Bastholt, P., 2000. Professional tennis (ATP Tour) and number of medical treatments in relation to type of surface. Medicine and Science in Tennis 5: 9.

Chapman, A.R., Vicenzino, B., Blanch and P., Hodges, P.W., 2007. Leg muscle recruitment during cycling is less developed in triathletes than cyclists despite matched cycling training loads. Experimental Brain Research 3: 503-518.

Chumanov, E.S., Schache, A.G., Heiderscheit, B.C. and Thelen, D.G., 2012. Hamstrings are most susceptible to injury during the late swing phase of sprinting. British Journal of Sports Medicine 46: 90.

Dowling, B.A. and Dart, A.J., 2005. Mechanical and functional properties of the equine superficial digital flexor tendon. Veterinary Journal 170: 184-192.

Gigante, A., Cesari, E., Busilacchi, A., Manzotti, S., Kyriakidou, K., Greco, F., Di Primio, R. and Mattioli-Belmonte, M., 2009. Collagen I membranes for tendon repair: effect of collagen fiber orientation on cell behavior. Journal of Orthopaedic Research 27: 826-832.

Gillis, C.L., 1997. Rehabilitation of tendon and ligament injuries. In: Proceedings of the 43rd Annual Convention of American Association of Equine Practitioners, Phoenix, AZ, USA, Dec 7-10, pp. 306-309.

Gillis, C.L., 2004. Soft tissue injuries: tendinitis and desmitis. In: Hinchcliff, K.W., Kaneps, A.J. and Geor, R.J. (eds.) Equine sports medicine and surgery: basic and clinical sciences of the equine athlete. Elsevier Limited, Philadelphia, PA, USA, pp. 412-432.

Gombatto, S.P., Klaesner, J.W., Norton, B.J., Minor, S.D. and Van Dillen, L.R., 2008. Validity and reliability of a system to measure passive tissue characteristics of the lumbar region during trunk lateral bending in people with and people without low back pain. Journal of Rehabilitation Research and Development 45: 1415-1429.

Guilak, F., Fermor, B., Keefe, F.J., Kraus, V.B., Olson, S.A., Pisetsky, D.S., Setton, L.A. and Weinberg, J.B., 2004. The role of biomechanics and inflammation in cartilage injury and repair. Clinical Orthopaedics and Related Research 423: 17-26.

Halsband, U. and Lange, R.K., 2006. Motor learning in man; a review of functional and clinical studies. Journal of Physiology 99: 414-424.

Hewett, T.E., Paterno, M.V. and Myer, G.D., 2002. Strategies for enhancing proprioception and neuromuscular control of the knee. Clinical Orthopaedics and Related Research 1: 76-94.

Lam, T., Wirz, M., Lunenburger, L. and Dietz, V., 2008. Swing phase resistance enhances flexor muscle activity during treadmill locomotion in incomplete spinal cord injury. Neurorehabilitation and Neural Repair 22: 438-46.

Lotz, J.C. and Ulrich, J.A., 2006. Innervation, inflammation, and hypermobility may characterize pathologic disc degeneration: review of animal model data. Journal of Bone and Joint Surgery American 88: 76-82.

Lukoschek, M., Boyd, R.D., Schaffler, M.B., Burr, D.B. and Radin, E.L., 1986. Comparison of joint degeneration models: surgical instability and repetitive impulsive loading. Acta Orthopaedica Scandinavica 57: 349-353.

Meershoek, L.S., Schamhardt, H.C., Roepstorff, L. and Johnston, C., 2001. Forelimb tendon loading during jump landings and the influence of fence height. Equine Veterinary Journal Suppl. 33: 6-10.

Piazza, S.J. and Delp, S.L., 1996. The influence of muscles on knee flexion during the swing phase of gate. Journal of Biomechanics 29: 723-733.

Rupp, J.D., Flannagan, C.A. and Kuppa, S.M., 2010. Injury risk curves for the skeletal knee-thigh-hip complex for knee-impact loading. Accident Analysis and Prevention 42: 153-158.

Sahrmann, S., 2002. Diagnosis and treatment of movement impairment syndromes, 1st ed. Mosby, St. Louis, MO, USA, pp. 1-7.

Sahrmann, S. and Bloom, N., 2011. Update of concepts underlying movement system syndromes. In: Sahrmann, S. (ed.) Movement system impairment syndromes of the extremities, cervical and thoracic spines. Elsevier, St. Louis, MO,USA, pp. 1-33.

Scholtes, S.A., Norton, B.J., Lang, C.E. and Van Dillen, L.R., 2010. The effect of within-session instruction on lumbopelvic motion during a lower limb movement in people with and people without low back pain. Manual Therapy 15: 496-501.

Sloet van Oldruitenborgh-Oosterbaan, M.M., Wensing, T.H., Barneveld, A. and Breukink, H.J., 1991. Work-load in the horse during vaulting competition. Equine Exercise Physiology 3: 331-336.

Spitznagel, T. and Ivens, R., 2011. Movement system syndromes of the thoracic spine. In: Sahrmann, S. (ed.) Movement system impairment syndromes of the extremities, cervical and thoracic spines. Elsevier, St. Louis, MO, USA, pp. 103-144.

Sterling, M., Jull, G. and Wright, A., 2001. The effect of musculoskeletal pain on motor activity and control. Journal of Pain 2: 135-145.

Van Dillen, L.R., McDonnell, M.K., Susco, T.M. and Sahrmann, S.A., 2007. The immediate effect of passive scapular elenation on symptoms with active neck rotation in patients with neck pain. Clinical Journal of Pain 23: 641-647.

Wakeling, J.M. and Horn, T., 2009. Neuromechanics of muscle synergies during cycling. Journal of Neurophysiology 101: 843-854.

Woo, S.L., Gomez, M.A., Sites, T.J., Newton, P.O., Orlando, C.A. and Akeson, W.H., 1987. The biomechanical and morphological changes in the medial collateral ligament of the rabbit after immobilization and remobilization. Journal of Bone and Joint Surgery American 69: 1200-1211.

6. Novel approaches for injury-prevention and monitoring of tendons and ligaments by means of ultrasound tissue characterization

H.T.M. van Schie[1,2]
[1]UTC Imaging, Kruisstraat 65, 6171 GD Stein, the Netherlands; [2]Institute of Sport, Exercise & Health, University College London, 170 Tottenham Court Road, London W1T 7HA, United Kingdom; hans.vanschie@utcimaging.com

Abstract

Repetitive loading of tendons and ligaments may lead to, initially a-symptomatic, matrix deterioration. The ultra-structural changes can be monitored by means of ultrasound tissue characterization (UTC), aiming at injury-prevention. In addition, the discrimination of stages of repair or developing pathology, like reactive, overstraining, inferior repair and degenerative stages may play a crucial role in the selection of appropriate treatment and guided rehabilitation, aiming at restoration of function, without relapses.

Keywords: healing, horse, lesions, rehabilitation, repair

Introduction

Injuries of flexor tendons and ligaments all too often threaten the athletic career as these elastic structures play a vital role in locomotor efficiency, acting as energy saving springs. This biomechanical function is based on the unique architecture consisting of a collagenous matrix that is 3-dimensionally organized into tendon bundles (fibres, fascicles).

Symptoms of tendinopathy are frequently only the tip of the iceberg; injuries may be due to single overloading, but more often the lesion is the result of gradual matrix deterioration due to repetitive overstraining which can remain unobserved for months or even years.

Also the reputedly bad healing tendency of injuries, leading to repair tissue that never completely regains its original characteristics, is a severe aggravating factor. Although horses may come back to their previous level of performance, in many cases relapses occur that may end the horse's athletic career or limit the performance to a lower level. Besides the inferior quality of repair, relapses are frequently also caused by the misinterpretation of the stage of the lesion and it's loading capacity during recovery.

Thus, for the optimal performance of the equine athlete a management aiming at early detection of exercise effects, staging of lesions and guided rehabilitation is prerequisite.

Ultrasonography (US) was introduced in the early 80's and appeared to have, like no other imaging technique, the potential to provide an inward view into the tendon's architecture (Rantanen, 1982). However, US measurements of the tendon's cross-sectional area or mean echogenicity have shown little benefits for monitoring of exercise effects and for evaluation of the stage of the injury and the quality of repair (Avella et al., 2009; Gillis et al., 1993; Van Schie et al., 2000). This is caused by the fact that US assessment is essentially subjective and poorly reproducible due to instrumental variables and transducer handling (Van Schie et al., 1999). Another confounding factor is that, as a consequence of limits of resolution, every US image is a mixture of structural reflections and interfering echoes: only relatively large structures, like secondary tendon bundles (fascicles), generate reflections, while smaller entities, such as fibrils and cells, will result in interference, each with their specific dynamics in real-time US which is not captured in still 2-dimensional US images (Van Schie et al., 2001).

Therefore, a method for computerized ultrasound tissue characterization (UTC) imaging was developed for the benefit of an objective evaluation of the integrity of the 3-dimensionally arranged collagenous matrix. UTC is based on standardized data-collection by means of an ultrasound probe that moves automatically along the tendon's long axis, collecting transverse images at even distances of 0.2 mm (Figure 1). In this way, a 3-D ultrasound data-block is created for tomographic visualization (in transverse, sagittal, coronal and 3-D coronal planes of view (Figure 2) and for the quantification of tendon

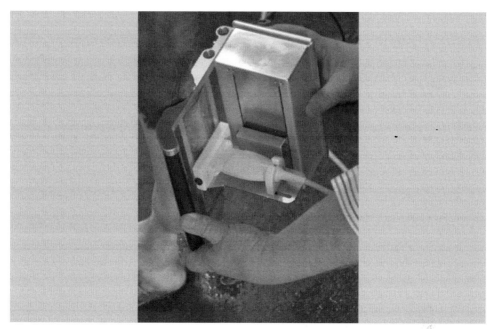

Figure 1. Standardised data-collection by means of ultrasound tissue characterization tracking device.

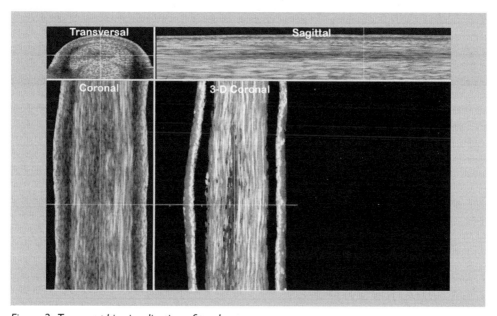

Figure 2. Tomographic visualisation of tendon structure.

matrix integrity. In this 3-D data-block dedicated UTC-algorithms can quantify the dynamics of echo-patterns in contiguous images which allows the discrimination of 4 different echo-types, related to size and integrity of structures in the matrix (Figure 3):

- echo-type I, generated by reflections at intact and aligned fascicles with axial diameter ≥0.35 mm (Figure 3A);
- echo-type II, generated by reflections at discontinuous, waving and/or swollen fascicles with axial diameter ≥0.35 mm (Figure 3B);
- echo-type III, generated by interfering echoes from matrix mainly consisting of fibrils with axial diameter <0.35 mm (Figure 3C);
- echo-type IV, generated by mainly amorphous matrix and fluid (Figure 3D).

Fundamental research on isolated tendons revealed that the ratios of these 4 echo-types are highly correlated with histo-morphological characteristics of tendon tissue, showing the discriminative power of UTC for tissue characterization (Van Schie *et al.*, 2001, 2009). Subsequently clinical research was started, with UTC as reliable tool

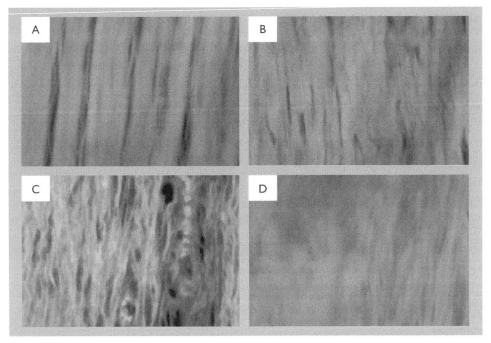

Figure 3. (A) Tissue generating echo-type I; (B) Tissue generating echo-type II; (C) Tissue generating echo-type III; (D) Tissue generating echo-type IV.

for staging of lesions, for monitoring tendon repair and for objective evaluation of therapeutic interventions like intra-tendinous injections of platelets rich plasma (PRP) and short-duration immobilisation (Bosch *et al.*, 2011; David *et al.*, 2011; Van Schie *et al.*, 2009). Furthermore, recent experiments, tested the hypothesis that cumulative effects of repetitive overstraining may lead to insidious deterioration of the tendon matrix and that UTC is sensitive enough to detect these changes long before clinical signs of a tendon injury become manifest (Docking *et al.*, 2012).

Clinical research

Clinical research was done in 4 different studies:
1. In young-mature horses (n = 18), both Warmblood and Standardbred (average 3.2 years of age) showing neither clinical nor ultrasonographic signs of tendinopathy in the superficial digital flexor tendon (SDF); SDF tendons in both front limbs were scanned. Tendon integrity was quantified by means of UTC in order to determine ratios of 4 echo-types representative for normal SDF tendon tissue. Furthermore intra- and inter-observer reliability was tested.
2. In young-mature horses, see study 1, standardised lesions were created surgically in SDF tendons in both front limbs and subsequently tendon repair was monitored, with UTC scans made at regular intervals, and matched with histomorphology of tissue specimen harvested post-mortem at 24 weeks (Bosch *et al.*, 2011; David *et al.*, 2011; Van Schie *et al.*, 2009).
3. In young racing Thoroughbreds (average 3.8 years of age; n = 13) in full race training the SDF tendons, showing neither clinical nor ultrasonographic signs of tendinopathy in both front limbs, were scanned within 8 h prior to race and 1, 2, and 3 days post-race (Docking *et al.*, 2012).
4. In high-performance horses (average 11.8 years of age) in disciplines showjumping (n = 14), dressage (n = 12) and eventing (n = 9) the SDF, deep digital flexor tendons (DDF), the inferior check ligaments (ICL) and the suspensory ligaments (SL) in front and hind limbs were monitored. Individual baseline values were determined by means of 3 UTC-scans made with monthly intervals and subsequently these horses were scanned regularly during training and competition for more than 2 years.

Major observations

Major observations were:
1. Normal SDF tendons in young-mature horses are characterised by 85-90% type I, 10-15% type II and less than 5% type III plus IV echoes (Bosch *et al.*, 2011; David *et al.*, 2011; Van Schie *et al.*, 2009).
2. Intra- and inter-observer reliability appeared to have intra-class correlation (ICC) ranging 0.92-0.98, indicative for the excellent reproducibility of UTC (Bosch *et al.*, 2011; David *et al.*, 2011; Van Schie *et al.*, 2009).
3. During monitoring of tendon repair several stages can be discriminated by UTC, and subsequently verified by means of post-mortem histology and biochemistry. This resulted in a time-schedule for non-intervened repair in 2-5 year old horses after single macro-trauma:
   a. initially, till 3 weeks post-injury, a rapid decrease of structure-related echo-types I plus II and a sharp increase of type IV was observed, related to an amorphous matrix and the presence of fluid during a stage called extension and demarcation of the lesion;
   b. from week 3 till 8 a significant increase of echo-type III and significant decrease of IV was observed, related to a fibrillar matrix becoming gradually more densely arranged during the fibrillogenesis stage;
   c. starting from weeks 9 till 12 a sharp increase of echo-types I and II was observed, indicative for fibrils getting organised into fascicles during early bundle formation stage;
   d. starting from weeks 13 till 24, there was continuing increase of type I, a gradual decrease of II and types III and IV tended to normal during so-called organization and remodelling stage.
   However, stages of repair do not always follow this timeframe; especially in older horses (>5 years of age) repair may take longer and lead to less quality of repair, most probably as a consequence of ageing and/or degeneration.
4. In race-horses subtle yet significant changes were observed in the SDF tendons at 1 and 2 days post-race, namely mild decrease of echo-type I and increase of echo-type II. These reactive changes returned to baseline, pre-race values within 3 days post-race. No significant increase of echo-types III and/or IV were observed (David *et al.*, 2011).

5. In high-performance horses in all disciplines the individual baseline values showed striking changes in echo-type, compared to those in young-mature horses, even without clinical signs and only limited increase of cross-sectional area (<15%). These changes were either a localised increase of echo-types II and III in the central core-region, or a more scattered increase of echo-types III and/or IV.

6. In 12-15% of high-performance horses the loading during competition led to changes (compared to pre-competition individual baseline values) within 4-7 days. This overstraining was characterised by significant increases of echo-type II, III and IV, however, only in some cases accompanied by short-duration clinical signs like moderate swelling and pain on palpation. Echo-types may return to baseline within 4-12 weeks or otherwise extensive changes may persist, leading to inferior repair (persistent increase of II and III) or degeneration (persistent increase of III and IV). These persistent changes frequently lead to intermittent flare-ups and ultimately even develop into a (partial) rupture.

Discussion

UTC can quantify ultra-structural integrity and it's excellent reproducibility is a prerequisite for monitoring of exercise effects and objective evaluation of therapeutic interventions like immobilization and regenerative therapies (PRP, stem cells). Post-injury repair does not always fit within the timeframe described; especially in older horses (>5 years of age) repair may take longer and lead to less quality of repair, most probably as a consequence of ageing and/or degeneration.

Short-duration changes observed on days 1 and 2 post-race are indicative for swollen and waving fascicles. These reactive changes usually return to baseline within 72 hours post-race, being the result of a cellular response to load with short-duration up-regulation of high-molecular hydrophilic proteoglycans. The swelling is due to an increase of inter-fibrillar ground substance, however without fibrillar disintegration and presence of free fluid in the inter-fascicular septa (endotenon; Docking *et al.*, 2012).

In striking contrast to young mature horses the SDF, DDF, ICL and/ or SL of high-performance horses, even without clinical signs, showed significant increases of echo-type II, III and/or IV. Based on previous fundamental research on isolated tendons a local increase of echo-types II and III, mainly in the central core-region could be related to the presence of fibrosis and inferior repair. Diffuse increase of echo-type II, III and/or IV can be related to overstraining with fibrillar disintegration and free fluid in the inter-fascicular septa, or otherwise be indicative for the presence of more persistent stages of inferior repair and degeneration.

During these experiments, the most striking observation was that SDF, DDF, ICL and SL in high-performance horses may show significant ultra-structural changes without symptoms. These observations on UTC confirm the hypothesis that clinical tendinopathy may have an insidious onset, being the result of a continuum inflicted by repetitive overstraining, initially without clinical signs. It is only at end-stage, when it comes to a tendon injury, that symptoms become manifest. In other words: symptoms are frequently only the tip of the iceberg and when symptoms develop the window of opportunity to achieve complete repair of ultra-structure and to restore full function is closed.

The following schedule for UTC-check-ups of high-performance horses, aiming at early detection of matrix deterioration, is recommended:
- measurement of individual baseline values of echo-types I, II, III and IV at 3 time-points;
  - prior to competition;
  - 4-7 days after competition;
    - if normalized (actually back to individual baseline values), than re-check with 8-12 week intervals;
    - if still abnormal, than re-check with 2-4 week intervals till baseline values.

It is concluded that repetitive loading of tendons and ligaments may lead to, initially a-symptomatic, matrix deterioration and that these ultra-structural changes can be monitored by means of UTC, aiming at injury-prevention. Furthermore, discrimination of stages of repair or otherwise developing pathology, like reactive, overstraining, inferior repair and degenerative stages has to play a crucial role in the selection of appropriate treatment and guided rehabilitation, aiming at restoration of function, without relapses.

References

Avella, C.S., Ely, E.R., Verheyen, K.L.P., Price, J.S., Wood, J.L. and Smith, R.K., 2009. Ultrasonographic assessment of the superficial digital flexor tendons of National Hunt racehorses in training over two racing seasons. Equine Veterinary Journal 41: 449-454.

Bosch, G., Van Weeren, P.R., Barneveld, A. and Van Schie, H.T., 2011. Computerised analysis of standardized ultrasonographic images to monitor the repair of surgically created core lesions in equine superficial digital flexor tendons following treatment with intratendinous platelet rich plasma or placebo. Veterinary Journal 187: 92-98.

David, F., Cadby, J., Bosch, G., Brama, P., Van Weeren, R. and Van Schie, H.T., 2011. Short-term cast immobilization is effective in reducing lesion propagation in a surgical model of equine superficial digital flexor tendon injury. Equine Veterinary Journal 44: 570-575.

Docking, S.I., Daffy, J., Van Schie, H.T. and Cook, J.L., 2012. Tendon structure changes after maximal exercise in the thoroughbred horse: use of ultrasound tissue characterisation to detect *in vivo* tendon response. Veterinary Journal 194: 338-342.

Gillis, C.L., Meagher, D.M., Pool, R.R., Stover, S.M., Craychee, T.J. and Willits, J., 1993. Ultrasonographically detected changes in equine superficial digital flexor tendons during the first months of race training. American Journal of Veterinary Research 54: 1797-1802.

Rantanen, N.W. 1982. The use of diagnostic ultrasound in limb disorders of the horse. A preliminary report. Journal of Equine Veterinary Science 2: 62-64.

Van Schie, H.T., Bakker, E.M., Jonker, A.M. and Van Weeren, R., 2000. Ultrasonographic tissue characterization of equine superficial digital flexor tendons by means of gray level statistics. American Journal of Veterinary Research 61: 210-219.

Van Schie, H.T., Bakker, E.M., Van Weeren, P.R. 1999. Ultrasonographic evaluation of equine tendons: a quantitative *in vitro* study of the effects of amplifier gain level, transducer-tilt and transducer-displacement. Veterinary Radiology and Ultrasound 40: 151-160.

Van Schie, H.T., Bakker, E.M., Jonker, A.M. and Van Weeren, R., 2001. Efficacy of computerized discrimination between structure-related and non-structure-related echoes in ultrasonographic images for the quantitative evaluation of the structural integrity of superficial digital flexor tendons in horses. American Journal of Veterinary Research 62: 1159-1166.

Van Schie, H.T., Bakker, E.M., Cherdchutham, W., Jonker, A.M., Van de Lest, C.H. and Van Weeren, P.R., 2009. Monitoring of the repair process of surgically created lesions in equine superficial digital flexor tendons by use of computerized ultrasonography. American Journal of Veterinary Research 70: 37-48.

7. The whole horse approach to equine rehabilitation: the myofascial view

V.S. Elbrønd
University of Copenhagen, Faculty of Veterinary Science, Department of Clinical and Animal Sciences, Section of Anatomy and Biochemistry, Grønnegårdsvej 7, 1870 Frederiksberg C, Denmark; vse@sund.ku.dk

Abstract

Overall full body models as the myofascial kinetic lines, which integrates functionally interrelated and integrated structures of the locomotion system, is necessary to better understand the collaborations in the locomotion system. In the myofascial kinetic lines the connective tissue plays a dominant role as well mechanical as in collaboration with the nervous system. The effect of a myofascia release is measurable in muscles with multi-frequency bioimpedance measurements, and it is shown to affect the health and function of the skeletal muscles.

Keywords: bioimpedance, locomotion, muscle, release, treatment

Introduction

Speaking of myofascia in the veterinary and equestrian world automatically directs the focus towards the locomotion system, which makes good sense. The generally accepted myofascial and biomechanical models, such as the bow-string theory (Slijper, 1946), the spring and recoil mechanism of the legs (McNeil Alexander, 2002; Wilson *et al.*, 2001, 2003) and the mechanical/passive stay apparatus (Gussekloo *et al.*, 2011; Wilson *et al.*, 2001), are frequently addressed when diagnosing, treating and rehabilitating horses. These models are limited to specific regions of the horse. None of them are integrated in a whole horse approach, and studies of a full body/whole horse model are rare to the best of our knowledge. However, new research and studies (Elbrønd and Schultz, 2014, 2015; Lesimple *et al.*, 2012; Rhodin *et al.*, 2009; Richter and Hebgen, 2009) show that the whole body approach is an essential inclusion for a comprehensive understanding of (1) the interaction of biomechanics; (2) how and why normal function, overuse and compensatory mechanisms interact; and (3) where and how to treat horses, when damage/problems occur.

Myers (2009) recently presented a model of the organization of the myofascial system in humans. This full body model comprised ten interacting anatomy trains, each with rows of functionally related myofascial structures with the connective tissue as the major component. The connective tissue was present in different conformations, such as fascia blades, tendons, peri- and epimysium, ligaments and periost. The lines were found to interact in a 3-dimensional network, so as to balance the body both whilst standing and in motion. The tensegrity model (Fuller, 1975) gives an impression of and explanation for why and how the structures in this 3-D network collaborate and affect each other. The tensegrity model takes into account only the interaction of the mechanical components (bones, muscles, connective tissue). The nervous system, however, performs the overall control and regulation of the body balance *via* the myofascial system. Several studies have presented the integration between the nervous systems and the fascia (Berlucchi and Aglioti, 2010, Stecco *et al.*, 2007; Van der Wal, 2009), but this interplay is far from fully understood, and new studies continue to provide us with a better overview and understanding of how this communication and collaboration works.

Humans, horses and a 'whole body approach'

Humans and horses are different in many ways. With regard to the locomotion system, the most striking differences are the posture, biped versus quadruped, the development/evolutionary variation of the legs and foot and the size and carriage of the neck and head. In common, though, is the continuous demand to maintain body balance in posture as well as in motion. The body always naturally seeks a posture or motion with the lowest demands with respect to energy consumption (Cavagna *et al.*, 1977). In the horse this means that the centre of gravity (COG) in a normally balanced and standing position loads $2/3$ of the body weight on the front part. Locomotion interrupts this balance and moves/pushes the COG and centre of motion (COM), with the result that the body continuously works to re-attain a body in balance by means of the easiest route and at the lowest level of energy consumption. Internal factors (pain, reduced activity in motion units, trauma, etc.) as well as external (saddle, bridle, equipment, different riders, different riding techniques, different sports) challenge the body balance of the horse (Eisersjö *et al.*, 2013; Greve and Dyson, 2014; Ramseier *et al.*, 2013). The nervous system plays an essential role in the perception and reflexion of these changes. A normal movement pattern is learned by experience and loaded into the memory of the nervous system as segmental and full body reflexes during repetitions of the movements/situations/challenges. The horses are continuously exposed to variations in and changes to their COG. The challenge then for the horses is to learn how to conserve and maintain the body balance under different conditions. Should it not prove strong enough to preserve an optimal body balance, then the horse will start to compensate and the body will once again choose the easiest way in which to perform/respond (again at the lowest level of energy consumption). Though the horse still has to perform and therefore the compensations force the body into conditions where some regions work inefficiently and others are overused (Eisersjö *et al.*, 2013; Greve and Dyson, 2014; Ramseier *et al.*, 2013, Van Weeren *et al.*, 2010). Continuous and repetitious compensations end up frequently in traumatic overuse of the trunk, extremities, neck, etc.

Local balance in the horse

In horses several local biomechanical models and balance systems are used and accepted in daily veterinary practice. The mechanical stay apparatus, the passive stay apparatus, the stomatognatic system, and the bow-string theory are just some of these. Research has enabled a more detailed understanding of the structural interactions associated with some of these models, but they should still be regarded as limited since they only present a fraction of the body. Moreover, no studies seem to examine any interactions between these models.

A full body approach

To get a full overview of the balance in a horse, a whole body approach is essential – and as such not only a whole body approach whilst standing, but also one in motion too. In addition a three dimensional approach has to be assessed to assure a full and informative interpretation of the biomechanics.

The human model of the anatomy trains (Myers, 2009) was transferred to horses by Elbrønd and Schultz (2014, 2015) resulting in the identification of equine myofascial kinetic lines. More than 22 horses were dissected and up to now 8 lines have been isolated. The horse lines (and the human trains) are long rows of functionally integrated and related anatomical structures, which balance the body in posture and locomotion. The major component being the fascia tissue (fascia sheets, tendons, ligaments, joint capsules, etc.), which assures the integrity from start to end and the continuity of these structures into an uninterrupted line in the body. Several of the equine kinetic lines/human anatomical trains span from head to toe. The lines obey specific rules such as their level/depth in the body, the direction of their collagen fibres and the functional interaction in the locomotion system. The lines in the horse were found to comprise many similar structures to those identified in the human trains. Moreover, the lines can be split into smaller local subunits.

To reflect the quadruped posture veterinary terminology was chosen to name the equine lines. Three of the isolated lines are engaged in shaping the superficial three-dimensional network of the body. These lines are: (1) superficial dorsal line (SDL); (2) superficial ventral line (SVL); and (3) lateral line (LL). These lines comprise structures involved in spinal flexion, extension and lateral flexion in relation to the horizontal plane. The three lines extend the previously mentioned bow-string theory (Slijper, 1946) and include the head, the neck and the hind limb (Figure 1). A full body 'bow and string' model is thereby introduced in the horse. The lines work individually or bilaterally in pairs depending on the posture and movement/gait. In the hind limb the three lines meet in the foot. The fascial structures integrate as part of the passive stay apparatus, the mechanical stay apparatus and the spring and recoil biomechanics in the foot. In the head the lines centre, attach and balance the mandible (point of rotation). This arrangement influences the functionality of the complex temporomandibular joint, over which a large part of the proprioception (up to 60%) is perceived. The joint is additionally the centre of the stomatognatic system (Vogt, 2011), in which the neck muscles and thorax sling are integrated.

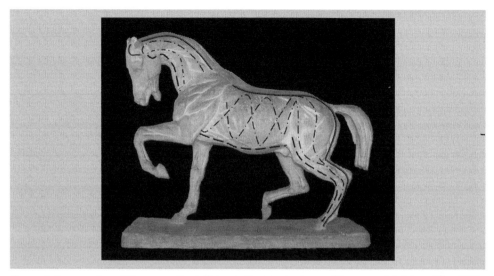

Figure 1. An overview of three myofascial kinetic lines in the horse. The superficial dorsal line (SDL, solid line), the superficial ventral line (SVL, dashed regular line) and the lateral line (LL, dashed and dotted line), which together make a three dimensional superficial network of the body. This network is involved in spinal flexion, extension and lateral flexion in relation to the horizontal plane.

Effects on and actions in the distal part of the hind limb influence structures throughout the full span of the line reaching the cervical and capital region and influencing the balance of the mandible. This gives quite a new perspective of the interplay that exists between the hindlimb and the head and (TMJ) and the line-structures 'in between'.

Additionally, two equine lines involved in spinal rotation and cross-coordination; (1) functional line (FL) and (2) spiral line (SPL) were dissected. Both lines represent a dorsal and a ventral part, which balance each other. The lines have two and three cross-overs, respectively, to the contralateral side and hereby provide an interaction between the right- and left-hand sides of the body. In the FL both the dorsal and ventral part cross the median plane once. The dorsal cross is situated in the lumbar fascia (Figure 2) and the ventral part in the prepubic and pubic region between the two *musculi gracili*. The FL creates a sling with a diagonal span between the axil of the front limb and the knee of the contralateral hindlimb. The FL is thereby involved in diagonal coordination and motion of the body.

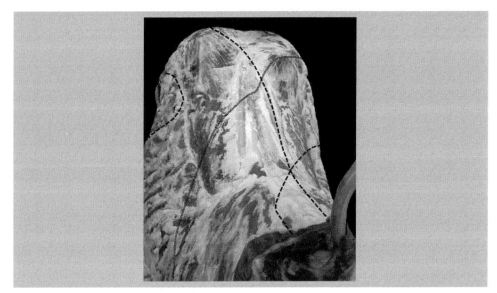

Figure 2. A cranio-dorsal aspect of the dorsum of a skinned horse. The course and two dorsal cross-overs of the two helical lines are presented. The functional line (FL, double line) and the spiral line (SPL, dashed line). The dorsal and straight part of the FL courses diagonally from right front to the left hind. The straight, dorsal part of the FL initiates from the left side of the head and runs along the left side of the back crossing over in the dorsal sacral ligaments to the right hindquarter and further on to the lateral side of the hock. The spiral part of the SPL initiates from the right side of the head and crosses over at the cervico thoracic junction. It continues under the abdomen to a ventral cross-over and becomes visible at the right flank wherefrom it directs towards the medial side of the hock. Here it fuses with the straight, dorsal part of the SPL.

The spiral line (SPL) follows a more complicated route as it originates and inserts on each side of the head. The line is divided into two parts: a straight part and a spiral part. The straight part is a mirror of the SDL from the head to the dorsal sacral region where it crosses over with the dorsal sacral ligaments (Figure 1) and continues into the profound hamstring muscles towards the lateral side of the hock. Distal to the *processus calcaneus* the spiral part contributes and completes the sling and from here it runs proximally and dorsolaterally with the distal hindlimb extensors and hip flexors to *tuber coxae* (Figure 2). From here it redirects into the fascia of the oblique abdominal muscles into a ventral cross over in the abdominal fascia and into the *musculus serratus ventralis* on the contralateral front limb. The third and dorsal cross-over is situated beneath the *ligamentum nuchae* (Figure 2) and from here the line runs in the dorsal neck to the head. The two helical lines (FL and SPL) interact uni- and bilaterally and balance the head, neck, trunk and hind limbs especially in cross-coordinated gaits such as walk, trot and canter, whereas in pace only the straight part of the spiral line dominates. FL and SPL additionally balance the hindlimbs with focus on pro- and supination of the hip joint, knee, stifle and foot.

Two horse armlines, a frontlimb protraction line (FLPL) and a frontlimb retraction line (FLRL), were dissected and isolated. Tom Myers (2009) additionally isolated two deep arm lines in the human. These lines have not yet been identified in the horse. One reason is the difficulties in isolation of the structures due to the strong and tight integrations of the fascia in the lower limb. Another reason is the obvious species differences in the front limb/arm motion patterns. The human arm has a considerable range of motion (ROM) with respect to ad- and abduction as well as rotation (pro- and supination). The horse front limb is designed to perform a stable pro- and retraction to establish and ensure speed, acceleration and deceleration. It is of great importance to mention the integration of the proximal part of the armlines into the two helical lines (FL, SPL) in both pro- and retraction motion. This serves to establish the functional interconnection between the front and hindlimbs and between the frontlimbs and trunk/neck.

A deep ventral line (DVL) was additionally dissected in the horse. This line was found to be very similar to the human line. The myofascial structures of the DVL included the hypaxial muscles and fascial structures of the neck and trunk, the diaphragm and the profound structures of the medial side of the thighs and the caudal side of the femur following the *musculus digitalis profundus* to the distal part of the hoof/foot. The line balances the body from inside and is involved in balancing all the external lines from head to foot/toe. Several structures of the line, e.g. *musculus psoas major et minor, musculus pectineus* and *musculi obturatorius* function as pelvic stabilisers by increasing the tonus/contraction, trying to re-establish a body balance. These internal contractions are difficult to approach but vital to understand and release in order to free the horse from any chronic imbalance.

Rehabilitation and myofascial kinetic lines

When the equine myofascial kinetic lines are in balance then the biomechanics are fully integrated and functioning optimally. Imbalances between the lines reflect conditions that impair the integration of the lines such as trauma, lameness, pelvic and sacral instabilities or reduced ROM, knee and stifle problems, somatic and visceral pains, scar tissue formation, etc. A whole body approach is therefore needed to re-establish a full body integrity and rebalance the myofascial kinetic lines.

Treatment of the myofascial lines can be done directly or indirectly as explained by Myers (2009). It is possible to approach traumatic or painful areas from a distance when treating other structures on the line. The full mechanism of this reaction is not yet clarified but the nervous system plays a dominant role. Quantification of fascia stiffness, tonus or contraction is difficult in domestic animals and can be hampered by the anatomy, such as: the fur, long or short, soft or stiff; the skin, thick or thin; as well as the presence of the cutaneous trunk musculature. These factors can represent significant obstacles in terms of precise measurement when using traditional methods such as a tonometer, electromyography and ultrasonography. Moreover, in order to obtain repeated measurements, a horses position should remain exactly the same, typically a relaxed position is ideal for the period required for measurement. This can from time to time be a challenge.

At the Veterinary Faculty of the University of Copenhagen, multi-frequency bioimpedance studies (mfBIA, measurements of the tissue's, e.g. resistance, centre frequency and membrane capacitance) in horses has improved our understanding of the post treatment reactions in myofascial structures to manual and mechanical fascia release. (Elbrønd, unpublished data; Harrison *et al.*, 2015). Our studies were designed to answer such questions as: (1) how can one quantify the effects of treatment; and (2) are the effects of treatment local and/or 'long distance', immediate and/or delayed, short term and/or persistent.

BIA measurements have been validated and widely accepted for use in humans, but over the last five to ten years they have also been used in domestic animals (horse and dog) (Bartels *et al.*, 2015;

Elbrønd, unpublished data; Harrison *et al.*, 2015; Riis *et al.*, 2013). Multi-frequency bioimpedance analysis therefore represents a unique method for obtaining essential information to evaluate the function and health of the locomotory system.

The mfBIA technique is non-invasive and fast, therefore making it a very suitable tool for use with animals. The bioimpedance instrument establishes a tiny current 800 mAmps at 256 frequencies over a range of 4 to 1000 KHz, performing 6 repeat measurements with a 1 sec interval. The animal contact is established ideally using pure platinum electrodes and conductive paste.

A typical multi-frequency bioimpedance analysis provides the user with information about bioelectrical components of the muscle tissue enabling an evaluation of the tissue composition and condition. The components are:

- *R – resistance*. The opposition to the flow of an alternating current through intra- and extracellular ionic solutions;
- *Xc – reactance*. Which is the delay in the passage of a current caused by the cell membranes and tissue interfaces (which provides information about the cellular size and health);
- *Mc*. The membrane capacitance (which provides information about cell activity and cell transport);
- *Ri*. The intracellular resistance (which has been found to be closely correlated to the cellular oxygen consumption at rest (Stahn *et al.*, 2008));
- *Re*. The extracellular resistance (which provides information about the degree of hydration in the extracellular/intercellular space and thereby registers oedema and muscle damage (Bartels *et al.*, 2015; Harrison *et al.*, 2015));
- *fc*, the centre frequency which quantifies the density of the muscle tissue (relaxed or contracted) (Bartels *et al.*, 2015; Harrison *et al.*, 2015).

Thus, repeated mfBIA measurements of the same spot on the same horse can be used to characterise and/or classify relative changes in hydration, tonus and cell health/damage especially in muscle tissue.

Manual myofascial release – a case study

A retired race horse with myofascial imbalance was treated using manual fascia release (long, soft stretch for 1-2 min) in the atlanto-occipital region (right side) and the region *tuber coxae* (left side), after a base-line mfBIA measurement had been taken, and the mfBIA recordings were then repeated at exactly the same sites 1 and 24 h after treatment. Results (Figure 3) showed major changes in the fc (centre frequency) of the *musculus obliquus internus abdominis sinister (m. obl. int. abd. sin.)*. After 1 h the *fc* fell from 60.9 to 51.6 kHz and after 24 h it fell again to 46.8 kHz (a normal resting centre frequency value). The reactance (*Xc*), impedance (Z) and resistance (R) values

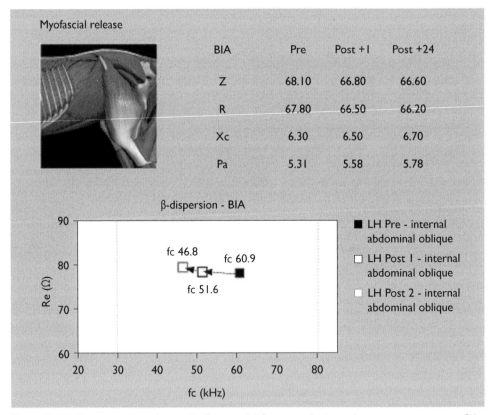

Figure 3. The figure presents the results from multi-frequency bioimpedance measurements of the m. obl. int. abd. sin. before, 1 and 24 h after a manual myofascial release. The fc (center frequency) values are presented in the diagram and a progress in the relaxation of the muscle is seen as a reduction in the delta fc values.

in contrast showed no significant changes over time compared with the baseline values as a result of fascia release treatment. The results observed reflect an increase in the muscle relaxation/reduction in muscle tone (*fc*) with fascia release treatment.

Mechanical myofascial release

Mechanical myofascial release was performed in a validation study of 6 horses with different myofascial imbalances. The horses were treated in two regions (right *regio atlanto-axialis- occipitalis* and right *regio coxae*) with mechanical multifrequent vibrations in exactly the same way. Multi-frequency bioimpedance was measured in *musculus splenius, musculus trapezius, musculus longissimus dorsi, musculus gluteus medius, m. obl. int. abd.* to follow the effect of treatment compared with baseline values at intervals of 1, 24 and 48 h post treatment. The centre frequency (*fc*) and the extra cellular resistance (Re) as well as the delta values between the left and right hand side were calculated. The results showed an immediate onset of a significant decrease in *fc* delta between right and left hand sides after 1 h, and a subsequent improvement over the next 24-48 h in relation to the baseline values. The overall results of the studies explain how the body works to re-establish a balance and muscular symmetry and tone post myofascial release treatment.

Conclusions

The biomechanics of the whole body of a horse is a complex model. The well-known biomechanical models, such as the bow-string, mechanical stay apparatus and stomatognatic system are regional and limited models. Overall full body models as the myofascial kinetic lines, which integrates the functionally interrelated and integrated structures of the locomotion system, is necessary to better understand the collaboration in the locomotion system. In the myofascial kinetic lines the connective tissue plays a dominant role, as well mechanical as in a collaboration with the nervous system. The effect of a myofascia release is measurable in muscles with multi-frequency bioimpedance measurements, and it is shown to affect the health and function of the skeletal muscles.

V.S. Elbrønd

Acknowledgements

I thank DVM R.M. Schultz for the collaboration with the dissections of the equine kinetic myofascial lines and comments to and corrections of the manuscript. I also want to thank my collegue Ass. Prof. Dr. Phil. A.P. Harrison for being a part of the collaboration with the bioimpedance studies, for using Figure 3, correcting and adjusting the manuscript. The studies of the kinetic myofascial lines in the horses were financially supported by 'The International Veterinary Chiropractic Association' (IVCA) and 'The Foundation for Promotion of Veterinary Science'.

References

Bartels, E.M., Sørensen, E.R., Harrison, A.P., 2015. Multi-frequency bioimpedance in human muscle assessment. Physiological Reports 3: e12354.

Berlucchi, G. and Aglioti, S.M., 2010. The body in the brain revisited. Experimental Brain Research 200: 25-35.

Cavagna, G.A., Heglund, N.C., Taylor, C.R., 1977. Mechanical work in terrestrial locomotion: two basic mechanisms for minimizing energy expenditure. American Journal of Physiology 233: R243-R261.

Eisersjö, M, Roepstorff, L., Weishaupt, M.A. and Egenvall, A., 2013. Movements of the horse's mouth in relation to horse-rider kinematic variables. Veterinary Journal 198: e33-e38.

Elbrønd, V.S. and Schultz, R.M., 2014. Myofascial kinetic lines in horses. Equine Veterinary Journal 46: 40.

Elbrønd, V.S. and Schultz, R.M., 2015. Myofascia – the unexplored tissue. Myofascial kinetic lines in horses, a model for describing locomotion using comparative dissection studies derived from human lines. Medical Research Archives. doi: http://dx.doi.org/10.18103/mra.v0i3.125.

Fuller, B., 1975. Synergetic. Macmillian, New York, NY, USA.

Greve, L. and Dyson, S., 2014. Saddle fit and management: an investigation of the association with equine thoracolumbar asymmetries, horse and rider health. Equine Veterinary Journal 47: 415-421.

Gussekloo, S.W.S., Lankester, J., Kersten, W. and Back, W., 2011. Effect of differences in tendon properties on functionality of the passive stay apparatus in horses. The American Journal of Veterinary Research 72: 474-483.

Harrison, A.P., Elbrønd, V.S., Riis-Olesen, K. and Bartels, E.M., 2015. Multi-frequency Bioimpedance in equine muscle assessment. Physiogical Measurements 36: 453-464.

Lesimple, C., Fureix, C., De Margerie. E., Sénèque, E., Menguy, H. and Hausberger, M., 2012. Towards a postural indicator of back pain in horses (*Equus caballus*). PLoS ONE 7: e44604.

McNeil Alexander, R., 2002. Tendon elasticity and muscle function. Review. Comparative Biochemistry and Physiology Part A 133: 1001-1011.

Myers, T., 2009. Anatomy trains – myofascial meridians for manual and movement therapists, 2nd ed. Churchill Livingstone, London, UK.

Ramseier, L.C, Waldern, N.M., Wiestner, T., Geser-von Peinen, K. and Weishaupt, M.A., 2013. Saddle pressure distributions of three saddles used for Icelandic horses and their effects on ground reaction forces, limb movements and rider positions at walk and tölt. Veterinary Journal 198: e81-e87.

Rhodin, M., Gómez Alvarez, C.B., Byström, A., Johnston, C., Van Weeren, P.R., oepstorff, L. and Weishaupt, M.A., 2009. The effect of different head and neck position on the caudal back and hindlimb kinematics in the elite dressage horse at trot. Equine Veterinary Journal 41: 274-279.

Richter, P. and Hebgen, E., 2009. Models of myofascial chains. In: Richter, P. and Hebgen, E. (eds.) Trigger points and muscle chains in osteopathy, 1st ed. Georg Thieme Verlag, Stuttgart, Germany, pp. 10-26.

Riis, K.H., Harrison, A.P., Riis-Olesen, K., 2013. Non-invasive assessment of equine muscular function: A case study. Open Veterinary Journal 3: 80-84.

Slijper, E.J., 1946. Comparative biologic-anatomical on the vertebral column and spinal musculature of mammals investigations, 1st ed. N.V. Noord-Hollandsche Uitgevers Maatschappij, Amsterdam, the Netherlands.

Stahn, A., Strobel, G. and Terblanche, E., 2008. VO_{2max} prediction from multi-frequency bioelectrical impedance analysis. Physiogical Measurements 29: 193-203.

Stecco, C., Gagey, O. and Belloni, A., 2007. Anatomy of the deep fascia of the upper limb. Second part: a study of innervation. Morphologie 91: 38-43.

Van der Wal, J.C., 2009. The architecture of the connective tissue in the musculoskeletal system: an often overlooked functional parameter as to proprioception in the locomotor apparatus. International Journal of Therapeutic Massage and Bodywork 2(4): 9-23.

Van Weeren, P.R., McGowan, C. and Haussler, K.K., 2010. Development of a structural and functional understanding of the equine back. Equine Veterinary Journal 42: 393-400.

Vogt, C., 2011. Zusammenhang zwischen Kiefergelenkemechanik und Ganz-körperstatik by Ros K. In: Vogt, C. (ed.) Lehrbuch der Zahnheilkunde beim Pferd, 1st ed., Schattauer GmbH, Stuttgart, Germany, pp. 35-39.

Wilson, A.M, Mc Guigan, M.P., Su, A. and Van den Bogert, A.J., 2001. Horses damp the spring in their step. Nature 414: 895-898.

Wilson, A.M., Watson, J.C. and Lichtwark, G.A., 2003. A catapult mechanism for rapid limb protraction. Nature 421: 35-36.

Expanded abstracts

8. Dimethylglycine supplementation in horses performing incremental treadmill exercise

K. de Oliveira[1]*, D.F. Fachiolli[1], M.J. Watanabe[2], D. Tsuzukibashi[3], C.M.M. Bittar[4], C. Costa[3], M.L. Poiatti[1] and P.R. de L. Meirelles[3]

[1]College of Animal Science, Experimental Campus of Dracena, Universidade Estadual Paulista 'Julio de Mesquita Filho' (UNESP), Rod Cmte. João Ribeiro de Barros, 651 km, Neighborhood: Bairro das Antas – Dracena, SP 17900-000, Brazil; [2]Department of Veterinary Surgery and Anesthesiology (DVSA), Faculty of Veterinary Medicine and Animal Science, Universidade Estadual Paulista 'Julio de Mesquita Filho', District Rubião Junior, s/n – Botucatu, SP 18618-970, Brazil; [3]Department of Animal Breeding and Nutrition (DABN), Faculty of Veterinary Medicine and Animal Science, Universidade Estadual Paulista 'Julio de Mesquita Filho' District Rubião Junior, s/n – Botucatu, SP 18618-970, Brazil; [4]Department of Animal Science, College of Agriculture 'Luiz de Queiroz', Universidade de São Paulo, Avenue Padua Dias 11, Piracicaba, SP 13418-900, Brazil; katia@dracena.unesp.br

Take home message

There was a significant effect of dimethylglycine supplementation over the reduction in the lactate concentration after the test exercise. Alterations of V_{200} (speed in which the horse reaches 200 heart beats/minute) and V_{LA4} (speed which corresponds to a blood lactate of 4 mmol/l) were not observed ($P > 0.05$), however there was a travelled distance elevation in the tests in function of the increase on the days of supplementation, by linear regression ($P < 0.05$) analysis.

Keywords: distance, heart rate, lactate, test

Introduction

The diverse available pathways for ATP production during exercise can be simultaneously utilised for energy production. The glucose stored in the form of glycogen in the muscles is utilised as fuel for ATP production, and in two main circumstances, lactate accumulation

A. Lindner (ed.) **Applied equine nutrition and training (ENUTRACO 2015)**
DOI 10.3920/978-90-8686-818-6_8, © Wageningen Academic Publishers 2015

occurs: (1) in situations where an oxygen deficiency occurs and (2) when there is the necessity of a greater production of energy per time unit which exceeds the capacity of the oxidative metabolism for ATP production (Boffi, 2007).

The lactate accumulation during physical activity is related to the beginning of fatigue, which compromises muscular contraction speed. Hence, studies have been developed in order to delay fatigue, being one of their lines, the utilization of ergogenic supplements. The main supplement evaluated for its efficacy in metabolic lactate removal over athletic performance in horses is trimethylglycine. This compound, known as betaine, is the dimethylglycine (DMG) precursor. Both supplements are the most utilised by horse trainers and owners (Warren *et al.*, 1999).

Friesen *et al.* (2007) described DMG as a glycine source for glutathione synthesis and it may act as a donor of methyl groups. Nonetheless, Levine *et al.* (1982) reported that the amount of lactic acid was significantly less in groups of horses consuming DMG and that this action could be a consequence of a greater activation of the pyruvate dehydrogenase enzyme. Warren *et al.* (1999) observed that the supplementation with the DMG precursor for 14 days, in untrained horses, influenced the lactate metabolism after exercise. Funari (2011) did not find beneficial effects for athletic performance in Arabian horses trained for endurance competition supplemented during 3 months with DMG at the dosage of 1.2 g/horse/day. The inconsistent effects of DMG supplementation described in literature might be attributable to different periods and dosages of supplementation too.

The objective of this study was to verify the effect of the DMG supplementation period in horses subjected to incremental exercise, on metabolic and physiologic parameters and indexes related to physical performance.

Material and methods

This study was certified by the Ethical Committee for Animal Use (ECAU), of the Animal Husbandry Course, São Paulo State University (UNESP), Dracena Campus, Brazil, under number 12/2013, according to the ethical principles of animal experimentation (funded by FAPESP 2013/13067-6). The authors have no conflicts of interest to declare.

The experiment was conducted at the School of Veterinary Medicine and Animal Husbandry of the São Paulo State University 'Júlio de Mesquita Filho', Campus Botucatu, SP. Four Arabian Purebred horses, three geldings and a female, on average eight years old and with a mean body weight (BW) of 340 kg, without controlled physical activity for at least two years, were used. Before beginning the experiment, the animals were clinically examined and considered healthy. They received an ivermectin-based dewormer, administered orally. During the whole experiment, the horses were kept in sand paddocks measuring 25×15 m, with no vegetal cover and water *ad libitum*.

The experimental delineation utilised was a Latin square 4×4, constituted by four periods of four weeks of evaluation, intercalated with four weeks of wash out periods, totalising four repetitions per treatment. The treatments consisted of periods of administration of a supplement with 30 g DMG (FastHorse – Marcolab, containing 85 g of DMG in 1 kg of product), administered orally, according to the manufacturer's recommendation. Therefore, the treatments were divided in a control group, without supplementation (S0), supplementation for 10 days (S10), supplementation for 20 days (S20) and supplementation for 30 days (S30). The supplementation with DMG during the evaluation period was initiated on the 20th day for the S10 group, on the 10th day for the S20 group, and on the first day for the S30 group. Plasma lactate concentration during and after exercise was measured, and the speed in which a horse reached 200 heart beats per minute (V_{200}), as well as a blood lactate of 4 mmol/l (V_{LA4}) in addition to the travelled distance (TD) determined; rectal temperature (RT) and heat rate (HR) before and after exercise were measured too.

In order to diminish possible factors that could interfere in the horses' metabolic and physiologic responses during the physical effort test, they were subjected to an adaptation period, where they were habituated to the treadmill exercise for 15 days (Mustang 2200 – Kagra, Fahrwangen, Switzerland) and to the nutritional management for 30 days. The horses' feeding was established to provide the minimal nutritional maintenance needs (NRC, 2007), resulting in the ingestion of dry matter (IDM) of 2.6% of the BW, in a relation of forage:concentrate of 66:34, respectively. The diet was composed of Tifton hay and commercial concentrate for equines (Proequi 13 Laminated – Guabi, Brazil) offered in three meals at 07, 13 and 19 hours. The mineral salt for equines (Centauro 80d – Guabi, Brazil) was offered in the amount of 90 g/animal/day always in the first meal of the day, during the whole experimental period. The DMG was offered to the horses in the last daily meal, mixed to the concentrate, in individual feeders and with consumption monitoring. In addition to this, the IDM was adjusted weekly, when necessary, in relation to the animals' BW.

On the day of the tests, the animals were prepared with an elastic belt with a heart rate transmitter (RS800CX – Polar, Kempele, Finland) and a blood collection system consisting of catheter (14 G Intracath – BD, São Paulo, Brazil), 60 cm extension tube (60 cm extension tube with LuerLock – Embramed, São Paulo, Brazil) and three-way stopcock. The exercise protocol was performed with the treadmill inclined to 6% and sequential phases of 2 minutes each in speeds of: 1.9 m/s (M1); 4.0 m/s (M2); 6.0 m/s (M3); 7.0 m/s (M4) and 8.0 m/s (M5); the treadmill was stopped when the horses could not maintain the speed even under humane stimulation. Samples of venous blood were collected via the system before beginning the exercise (M0) and during the last 20 seconds of each speed while the horse was exercised. Blood samples were also collected at time 3 (M6), 5 (M7), 10 (M8), 15 (M9), 30 (M10), 60 (M11), through the collection system; and 90 (M12), 120 (M13) and 360 (M14) minutes after the end of the exercise, by jugular venipuncture.

The blood samples were collected in sodium fluoride tubes and immediately packed in a Styrofoam container with shaved ice (Silva et al., 2012). The plasma was obtained by sample centrifugation at $1,087 \times g$ per 4 min. (Combate Centrifuge; Celm, Alphaville, Brazil), and packed in plastic tubes with 1 ml capacity, identified and stored in freezer at -16 °C temperature. The plasma lactate concentrations were determined by automatic equipment for clinical biochemistry (SBA-200 – Celm, Alphaville, Brazil) at the Animal Metabolism Laboratory of the 'Luiz de Queiroz' Superior School of Agriculture – USP – Piracicaba, SP, Brazil.

The V_{200} was calculated by linear regression between the HR values obtained in the last 20 seconds of each speed versus the exercise speed in m/s, in the moments where HR elevation proportional to the exercise speed was observed, using the Excel program (Soares, 2008). The V_{LA4} was calculated through exponential regression analysis of the relation between the plasma lactate concentrations and exercise speed. The travelled distance (m) was recorded for each horse after the conclusion of the treadmill effort test.

The horses' metabolic, physiologic and performance variables were subjected to variance analysis in SAS (Cary, NC, USA) and the comparisons between the averages were performed by the Tukey test to a 5% of significance (SAS, 2009). The breakdown of the degrees of freedom in orthogonal polynomials (Cohran and Cox, 1967) was accomplished. The coefficient of variation was utilised as a measurement of data dispersion.

Results

The DMG supplementation during 30 days significantly decreased the lactate concentration after the test exercise at M9, M10 and M11 in comparison with the control group (Table 1). This study identified a significant linear effect of the increased number of days with DMG supplementation (DS) on the reduction of the plasma lactate concentration during the effort test at M4 (Lactacidemia M4 = 11.9593 − 0.11695 × DS, R^2 = 0.29, P < 0.05) and M5 (Lactacidemia M5 = 13.5705 − 0.0727 × DS, R^2 = 0.38, P < 0.05).

Differences among treatment groups on V_{200} and V_{LA4} (Table 2) were not observed (P > 0.05), but there was an elevation on the tests' travelled distance in function of the number of days of supplementation by means of linear regression analysis (TD = 2,614.72 + 28.96 × DS, R^2 = 0.26, P < 0.05). Based on Table 3 data analysis, it was verified that there was no effect from the DMG supplementation in horses on the HR (P > 0.05) and there was only a significant difference between treatments for RT after exercise, where the supplementation for 30 days resulted in values statistically superior to the control group.

Table 1. Mean plasma lactate concentration during and post exercise tests in horses supplemented with dimethylglycine (DMG).

Moments (M)		Days of DMG supplementation[1]				CV[2] (%)
		0	10	20	30	
During exercise	M0 (rest)	0.69	1.45	1.39	1.34	38.20
	M1 (1.9 m/s)	0.81[a]	1.53[ab]	1.95[b]	2.00[b]	43.29
	M2 (4 m/s)	2.50	2.77	3.03	2.67	27.52
	M3 (6 m/s)	7.20	6.77	6.51	5.15	31.86
	M4 (7 m/s)	11.97	10.63	9.89	8.32	24.66
	M5 (8 m/s)	13.89	12.47	11.91	11.66	10.91
Post exercise	M6 (3 min)	13.45	13.50	13.38	13.03	2.87
	M7 (5 min)	13.28	13.35	13.25	12.98	3.54
	M8 (10 min)	13.33	13.28	13.03	12.68	4.20
	M9 (15 min)	13.10[b]	13.13[b]	12.33[ab]	11.68[a]	7.57
	M10 (30 min)	11.20[ab]	11.45[b]	9.85[ab]	8.75[a]	18.62
	M11 (1 h)	6.43[b]	5.08[ab]	3.70[a]	3.83[a]	37.49
	M12 (1 h 30 min)	2.83	1.73	1.50	1.68	49.66
	M13 (2 h)	1.33	1.15	1.55	1.33	29.77
	M14 (6 h)	0.68	1.00	1.63	0.38	49.17

[1] Mean values with superscript different letters on the same line differ amongst themselves by the Tukey test (P<0.05).
[2] CV = coefficient of variation.

Table 2. Mean values of the performance indexes in horses supplemented with dimethylglycine (DMG) subjected to an incremental treadmill test.

Variable[1]	Days of DMG supplementation					CV[2] (%)
	0	10	20	30	Average	
V_{200} (m/s)	4.5	4.6	4.7	4.8	4.7	8.94
V_{LA4} (m/s)	4.8	4.7	4.6	5.1	4.8	16.67
TD (m)	2,596	2,924	3,211	3,466	3,049	27.72

[1] V_{200} = speed in which the horse reaches a HR of 200 bpm; V_{LA4} = speed corresponding to a 4 mmol/l plasma lactate; TD = travelled distance.
[2] CV = coefficient of variation.

Table 3. Mean values of the physiologic parameters in horses supplemented with dimethylglycine (DMG) subjected to an incremental treadmill test.

Variable[1]	Days of DMG supplementation[2,3]								CV[4] (%)
	0		10		20		30		
	Pre	Post	Pre	Post	Pre	Post	Pre	Post	
HR (bpm)	34.0	89.5	37.0	86.3	37.0	87.8	35.0	89.3	13.54
RT (°C)	36.9	37.8[a]	37.1	38.3[ab]	37.1	38.4[ab]	37.2	38.7[b]	10.24

[1] HR = heart rate (beats per minute); RT = rectal temperature.

[2] Pre = evaluation performed before the test, Post = evaluation performed after the test.

[3] Averages with different superscript letters on the same line differ amongst themselves by the Tukey test ($P<0.05$).

[4] CV = coefficient of variation.

Conclusions

The supplementation with 30 g/day of a dimethylglycine-based product during one month reduced plasma lactate and increased the travelled distance during a treadmill incremental test in horses. Shorter periods of supplementation had no effects.

References

Boffi, F.M., 2007. Metabolismo enerjéticos y exercicio. Fisiologia del ejercicio en equinos. Inter-médica Editorial, Buenos Aires, Argentina.

Cohran, W.G. and Coc, G.M., 1967. Experimental designs. John Wiley and Sons, New York, NY, USA.

Friesen, R.W., Novak, E.M., Hasman, D. and Innis S.M., 2007. Relationship of dimethylglycine, choline, and betaine with oxoproline in plasma of pregnant women and their newborn infantis. Journal of Nutrition 137: 2641-2646

Funari, S., 2011. Avaliação da Suplementação com Dimetilglicina sobre o Desempenho Atlético de Cavalos de Enduro. Dissertação (Mestrado em Ciências) – Faculdade de Medicina Veterinária e Zootecnia, Universidade de São Paulo, Pirassununga.

Levine, S., Myhre, G., Smith, G. and Burns, J., 1982. Effect of a nutritional supplement containing N,N-dimethylglycine (DMG) on the racing standard bred. Equine Practice 4:1-3.

National Research Council (NRC), 2007. Nutrients requirements of horses. Washington, DC, USA.

Silva, M.A.G., Gomide, L.M.W., Bernadi, N.S. and Dias D.P.M., 2012. Equilíbrio ácido-base em eqüinos da raça quarto de milha antes e após a prova dos três tambores. Revista de Educação Continuada em Medicina Veterinária e Zootecnia 10: 84.

Soares, O.A.B., 2008. Comparação de diferentes métodos lactacidêmicos e glicêmicos de determinação do limiar anaeróbio em equinos. Dissertação (Mestrado) – Universidade Estadual Paulista, Faculdade de Ciências Agrárias e Veterinárias, Jaboticabal.

Statistical Analysis System (SAS), 2000. SAS user´s: guide statistics. SAS, Cary, NC, USA.

Warren, L.K., Lawrence, L.M. and Thompson, K.N., 1999. The influence of betaine on untrained and trained horses exercising to fatigue. Journal of Animal Science 77: 677-684.

9. Gymnastic training and dynamic mobilization work in therapy horses improve the stride and epaxial musculature quality

K. de Oliveira[1]*, R.V.G. Soutello[1], R. da Fonseca[1], C. Costa[2], P.R. de L. Meirelles[2], D.F. Fachiolli[1] and H.M. Clayton[3]
[1]College of Animal Science, Experimental Campus of Dracena, Universidade Estadual Paulista 'Julio de Mesquita Filho' (UNESP), Rod Cmte. João Ribeiro de Barros, 651 km, Neighborhood: Bairro das Antas – Dracena, SP 17900-000, Brazil; [2]Department of Animal Breeding and Nutrition (DABN), Faculty of Veterinary Medicine and Animal Science, Universidade Estadual Paulista 'Julio de Mesquita Filho' District Rubião Junior, s/n, Botucatu, SP 18618-970, Brazil; [3]Sport Horse Science, LLC, 3145 Sandhill Road, Mason, MI 48854, USA; katia@dracena.unesp.br

Take home message

Overtracking at walk ($P < 0.05$) was observed only in horses subjected to gymnastic work (GYM), in which the difference between the final and initial evaluations for the tracking distance at walk was 16.73 cm ($P < 0.05$). Significant hypertrophy of *musculus multifidus* occurred in the dynamic mobilization exercises and GYM groups, resulting in final mean values of 10.38 and 10.86 cm^2, respectively.

Keywords: bending, hippotherapy, flexion, locomotion, mobilization, pain, physical activity

Introduction

Hippotherapy is a form of therapy which uses horses as a treatment instrument for practitioners to treat individuals who have disabilities or special needs. Due to the therapeutic function in continuing sessions, associated with the lack of supportive physical activity, hippotherapy horses may become susceptible to muscular pain (Rosa, 2006; Silva *et al.*, 2012). This may have similar origin to the muscular pain experienced by human labourers, who, due to overloading or repetitive movements and lack of exercise, become susceptible to obesity, back pain and articular mobility problems (Allender *et al.*, 2006).

Rosa (2006) reported that during a therapeutic riding session, the horse is subjected to the patient's different body weights, postural deviations, and body imbalances. This study identified a negative change on the horse's stride quality in situations in which the subjects presented special characteristics, such as pelvic misalignment and excessive body weight. It is known that lumbar pain interferes with the horse's stride quality (Janura *et al.*, 2007) and is related to epaxial muscle damage, mainly affecting the *musculus multifidus* (McGowan *et al.*, 2003).

For a long time, gymnastic training in humans has contributed to the prevention of occupational diseases and rehabilitation. Gymnastic training can be performed by stretching and/or muscular strengthening exercises. Muscular stretching is a vital component in functional restoration. Its objective is to control the physiologic effects from deconditioning and to start to re-establish the normal amplitude of movement (Neblett *et al.*, 2003). Likewise, the dynamic mobilization exercises presented in the study by Stubbs *et al.* (2011) stimulated activation of the dorsal musculature which is used to stabilize the intervertebral joints, specifically *musculus multifidus*, resulting in its hypertrophy.

Stride quality is important for enabling therapy horses to perform the three-dimensional locomotor movements efficiently (Svoboda *et al.*, 2011), but dorsal stretching (Clayton, 2004) and strengthening of the abdominal and pelvic musculature (Higgins, 2009a) are fundamental pre-requisites often neglected by researchers in this area. According to Dvorakova *et al.* (2009), the combined action of the dorsal and ventral musculature of horses influences the three-dimensional movement. Thus, the therapy horse must have an extreme movement potential for the patient to receive a quality treatment, that accelerates the therapeutic and rehabilitation process. In this sense, our objective was to evaluate the efficacy of gymnastic training and dynamic mobilisation exercises in therapy horses, on stride quality and epaxial musculature, through linear kinematic analysis and muscular biometry.

Material and methods

This study was approved by the Ethical Committee for the Use of Animals (ECUA), of the Animal Husbandry Course, São Paulo State University (UNESP), Dracena Campus, Brazil, under protocol number 36/2012, in accordance with the ethical principles of animal experimentation.

The study was conducted in the APAE rural hippotherapy center, located in the town of Dracena – SP. The inclusion criteria for horses were that the horses showed no visible lameness and no signs or symptoms compatible with musculoskeletal lesions, the horses were habituated to hippotherapy sessions for three years and the horses were in regular work. This selection resulted in the utilization of nine cross-bred therapy horses, with an average age of 16 years and average body weight of 450 kg. The experimental design was completely randomized, with three treatments, resulting in three repetitions per treatment. The treatments were: control group, i.e. sedentary (SED), without physical activity performance, a group in which the horses performed dynamic mobilization exercises (DME) and a group in which the horses performed gymnastic work (GYM).

The total experiment lasted three months, during which time the horses performed the exercises under the supervision of a trained professional three times weekly, always performed on foot and guided by the halter. The physical activity performed with the horses obeyed the treatment designations, with exception of the SED group, which did not perform any type of physical activity. Therefore, the DME group exercises were designed to activate the spinal stabilizing muscles, following the description from papers by Stubbs and Clayton (2008) and Stubbs *et al.* (2011). Thus, the DME exercise consisted of three cervical flexion exercises, a cervical extension exercise and three lateral cervical bending exercises (performed to the right and left sides), in a total of ten mobilizations. Each mobilization exercise was repeated five times for each exercise session fusing treats in order to entice the horses to the desired positions.

The GYM group performed dynamic mobilization exercises together with exercises to recruit and strengthen the abdominal muscles and the pelvic stabilizing. The abdominal strengthening was performed by backing up, spinning and pelvic inclination exercises and the pelvic stabilizing muscles were strengthened by stepping over obstacles at walk. The muscular strengthening exercises followed the detailed description contained in the papers by Higgins (2009a,b). The backing up was performed in a single series of 10 consecutive steps in a straight line; the spinning was performed with the aid of a barrel, in a total of three repetitions per side per session; the pelvic inclination was gently performed by a reflex point localized between the *biceps femoris* and *semitendinosus* (five repetitions per session) and the obstacle exercise was performed by walking over a pole raised to a height of 40 cm for a period of 10 minutes; in clockwise and anticlockwise directions.

The experimental variables were recorded during two evaluations: the first performed before the beginning of the exercises period (day 0) and the second obtained after performing the activity for three months (day 90). The variables related to linear kinematics, such as stride length (SL) and tracking distance (TD), were measured in order to evaluate stride quality and to verify pelvic limb engagement. The biometric evaluations of the muscles were supported by monitoring the size of *longissimus dorsi* and *musculus multifidus*, to evaluate the epaxial musculature development.

In order to perform the evaluations, a lane 8 m long and 2 m wide was built on a sand track. Prior to the evaluations, the horses were subjected to a warm up session for 15 minutes at walk guided by the halter, and then taken to the sand lane for measurement (Janura *et al.*, 2010). The horses passed through the lane three times at walk, at an average speed of 1.3 m/s, with the speed being monitored by a photocell (Janura *et al.*, 2010). Hence, the displacement of the horses at walk was analysed three times, during a minimum of three repetitions, and the test with the speed nearest to 1.3 m/s was selected for the evaluations (Schils *et al.*, 1993). The horses' movements were captured at 25 Hz by a video camera that was perpendicular to and 8 m from the evaluation track (Hill and Cook, 2010).

The SL was determined by the distance between successive ground contacts of the left forelimb and the TD was the distance between the hoofprints of the left hindlimb and left forelimb. The value was designed positive if the hindlimb stepped ahead of the ipsilateral forelimb (over-tracking) or negative if the hindlimb stepped behind the ipsilateral forelimb (under-tracking) the hindlimb stepped into the hoofprint of the forelimb, the tracking distance was zero, and the horse was said to be tracking up tracking up (Clayton, 2004).

The evaluations of the horses' muscular development were performed ultrasonographically using Pie Medical Scanner 200 VET (Pie Medical, Maastricht, the Netherlands) equipment in real time, with a 3.5 MHz transducer 13 cm in length. The ultrasographic images were obtained by the same qualified professional and on the animal's left side. Three measurements from each muscular variable were collected as recommended by Stubbs *et al.* (2011). The *longissimus dorsi* (LD) measurement was performed at the level of the two last ribs, according to D'Angelis *et al.* (2005), with the animal standing in a straight position with relaxed muscles. The *musculus multifidus* (MM) image was obtained at the level of the fifth lumbar vertebra (Stubbs *et al.*, 2011). The LD thickness determination and the MM cross-sectional area were obtained by the manufacturer's software.

The standard deviation was used to express the variability. The variables related to linear kinematics and muscular biometry were subjected to the variance analysis using SAS (SAS, 2000). When significant differences between means were detected, the post hoc Tukey test was used. The variables obtained before and after the exercise program within the same horse, were compared through the paired t-test. The statistical tests used a 5% probability.

Results

Horses subjected to gymnastics training took longer strides at walk than horses in the sedentary and dynamic mobilization groups ($P<0.05$) (Table 1). SL average value at walk was 136 cm during the experimental period following all treatments, maintaining a constant speed at walk of 1.3 m/s in both evaluations.

Overtracking at walk ($P<0.05$) was observed only in horses subjected to GYM, in which the difference between the final and initial evaluation for the tracking distance at walk was 16.73 cm (Table 2). The TD at walk remained unaltered ($P>0.05$) between the initial and final measurement for the horses from the SD (average of -14.09 cm) and

Table 1. Difference between the initial and final measurement of stride length (SL) and tracking length (TL) in horses submitted to different treatments.

Variable (cm)	Treatments[1,2]			P-value	Standard deviation
	SD	DME	GYM		
SL at walk	0.67[b]	2.33[b]	10.67[a]	0.0004	4.82
TL at walk	1.83[b]	1.86[b]	16.73[a]	0.0002	7.65

[1] SD = sedentary; DME = dynamic mobilization exercise; GYM = gym work.
[2] Means with different superscript letters in the same line differ by Tukey test (P<0.05).

Table 2. Mean values of final and initial evaluations of tracking length in horses submitted to different treatments.

Treatments	Tracking length (cm)		P-value[1]	Standard deviation
	Initial	Final		
Sedentary	-15.00	-13.17	0.6318	4.01
Dynamic mobilization	-8.30	-6.44	0.2910	1.96
GYM work	-11.43	5.30	0.0010	3.07

[1] Paired t-test.

DME (average of -7.37 cm) groups (Table 2), showing that the horses' hindlimbs contacted the ground 14 and 7 cm behind the forelimbs.

In the current study, no LD hypertrophy ($P > 0.05$) was observed, even though there was a numeric increment in all the experimental groups (Table 3). However, dynamic mobilisation or exercises associated with muscular strengthening (GYM) in hippotherapy horses were able to significantly increase the cross-sectional area of the deep stabiliser muscles of the horse's back ($P < 0.05$) (Table 3). Significant hypertrophy of MM occurred in the DME and GYM groups, resulting in final mean values of 10.38 and 10.86 cm^2 respectively (Table 4).

Table 3. Difference between the initial and final measurement of the epaxial muscles in horses submitted to different treatments.

Variable	Treatment[1,2]			P-value	Standard deviation
	SD	DME	GYM		
Longissimus dorsi (cm)	2.38	3.98	2.43	0.0685	2.91
Musculus multifidus (cm²)	-0.55[b]	3.55[a]	3.78[a]	0.0040	6.48

[1] SD = sedentary; DME = dynamic mobilization exercise; GYM = gym work.
[2] Means with different superscript letters in the same line differ by Tukey test ($P<0.05$).

Table 4. Average values of initial and final valuation of musculus multifidus in horses submitted to different treatments.

Treatments	Musculus multifidus (cm²)		P-value[1]	Standard deviation
	Initial	Final		
Sedentary	7.57	7.02	0.9083	2.17
Dynamic mobilization	6.83	10.38	0.0215	3.15
GYM work	7.08	10.86	0.0407	4.37

[1] Paired t-test.

Conclusions

Gymnastic training, performed three times weekly, may become an important tool for horses used in hippotherapy programs, in order to improve stride quality and to promote the hypertrophy of the *musculus multifidus*.

References

Allender, S., Cowburn, G. and Foster, C., 2006. Understanding participation in sport and physical activity among children and adults: a review of qualitative studies. Health Education Research 21: 826-835.

Clayton, H.M., 2004. The dynamic horse. Sport Horse Publications, Mason, OH, USA.

D'Angelis, F.H.F., Ferraz, G.C. and Boleli, I.C., 2005. Aerobic training but not creatine supplementation alters the gluteus medius muscle. Journal of Animal Science 83: 579-585.

Dvorakova, T, Janura, M. and Svoboda, Z., 2009. The influence of the leader on the movement of the horse in walking during repeated hippotherapy sessions. Acta Universitatis Palacki Olomucensis Gymnica 39: 43-50.

Higgins, G., 2009a. How your horse moves. 1st ed. David & Charles Book, Cincinnati, OH, USA.

Higgins, G., 2009b. Pilates and stretching. 1st ed. Horse Inside Out Publication, Cincinnati, OH, USA.

Hill, C. and Crook, T., 2010. The relationship between massage to the equine caudal hindlimb muscles and hindlimb protraction. Equine Veterinary Journal 42: 638-687.

Janura, M., Dvorakova, T. and Peham, C., 2010. The influence of walking speed on equine back motion in relation to hippotherapy. Veterinary Medicine Austria 97: 1-5.

McGowan, C., Stubbs, N., Hodges, P. and Jeffcott, L., 2007. Back pain in horses – epaxial musculature. Rural Industries Research and Development Corporation, November 2007.

Neblett, R., Gatchel, J.R. and Mayer, G.T., 2003. A clinical guide to surface-EMG – Assisted stretching as an adjunct to chronic musculosketal pain rehabilitation. Applied Psychophysiology and Biofeedback 28: 147-160.

Rosa, L.R., 2006. Biomechanical analysis of a horse therapy: the interference of body weight and posture of the symmetry of the quality of the practitioner step horse. In: XII Congresso Brasileiro de Equoterapia, Brasília, Brazil, pp. 218-229.

Schils, S.J., Greer, N.L., Stoner, L.J. and Kobluk, C.N., 1993. Kinematic analysis of the equestrian – walk, posting trot and sitting trot. Human Movement Sciences 12: 693-712.

Silva, M.N.G., Folchini, N.P., Mistieri, M.L.A., Freitas, G.S.R., Sodré, L.A.D. and Duarte, C.A., 2012. Survey of disorders occurring in horses used in hippotherapy in period 2006 a 2010 in Uruguaiana-RS. Revista Brasileira de Ciência Veterinária 19: 139-143.

Statistical Analysis System (SAS). SAS user´s: guide statistics. SAS, Cary, NC, USA.

Stubbs, N.C. and Clayton, H.M., 2008. Activate your horses core. Sport Horse Publications, Mason, OH, USA.

Stubbs, N.C., Kaiser, L.J., Hauptman, J. and Clayton, H.M., 2011. Dynamic mobilization exercises increase cross sectional area of *musculus multifidus*. Equine Veterinary Journal 43: 522-529.

Svoboda, Z., Dvořáková, T. and Janura, M., 2011. Does the rider influence the horses movement in hippotherapy? Acta Universitatis Palackianae Olomucensis. Gymnica 41: 37-41.

10. Effect of an eventing season on V_{LA2} and V_{LA4} of Brazilian Sport Horses

B. Gonçalves de Souza[1], F. Gomes Ferreira Padilha[1*], F. Queiroz de Almeida[2] and A.M. Reis Ferreira[1,3]
[1]Programa de Pós Graduação em Clínica e Reprodução Animal, Universidade Federal Fluminense, Brazil; [2]Universidade Federal Rural do Rio de Janeiro, Brazil; [3]Setor de Anatomia Patológica Veterinária, Universidade Federal Fluminense, Brazil; felipe_padilha@yahoo.com.br

Take home message

V_{LA2} and V_{LA4} decreased after 22 weeks of an eventing season, but the difference was not significant ($P > 0.05$).

Keywords: competition, exercise test, lactate, season training

Introduction

In Eventing, there is no racial predominance linked to specific characteristics of this equestrian sport (Marlin *et al.*, 2001). The study of equine exercise physiology has been decisive to understand how the body of these athletes responds to exercise and how these responses are modified through different training protocols (Snow and Valberg, 1994). Such studies often involve the measurement of blood or plasma lactate concentrations before and during physical effort (Lindner and Boffi, 2007). According to Lindner (2000), blood lactate concentration is the variable that has shown most often a good relationship with the competitive performance of athletic horses, and because of its easy measurement is frequently used to evaluate their conditioning too. The workload of horses training and competing in eventing may cause deleterious effects on their athletic performance leading to poorer results. The aim of this work was to evaluate the effect of an eventing season on V_{LA2} and V_{LA4} of Brazilian Sport Horses.

A. Lindner (ed.) **Applied equine nutrition and training (ENUTRACO 2015)**
DOI 10.3920/978-90-8686-818-6_10, © Wageningen Academic Publishers 2015

B. Gonçalves de Souza et al.

Material and methods

This experiment was conducted in the Horse's Performance Evaluation Laboratory (LADEq), located at the Brazilian Army Cavalry School, Rio de Janeiro, Brazil. Seven Brazilian Sport Horses were used, aged from six to twelve years, four males and three females, in training for eventing competitions. The horses were stabled in individual stalls and fed with Coast Cross hay (*Cynodon dactylon*), commercial concentrate, 50 g of mineral salt and free access to water. The day before the tests, the horses were worked lightly, and the day after the effort test, the horses were kept in stalls at rest.

The training consisted of 90 minutes of daily exercise for six days per week, divided into flatwork, aerobic conditioning and jumping (on both track and natural obstacles), two days each. The seventh day was used to rest the horses, when they were walked for 10 minutes. The training protocol lasted for 22 weeks. The horses competed within 8-week intervals, totalizing three eventing competitions. The tests were conducted before and after the competitive season of 22 weeks.

The preparation of the animals for testing began with the antiseptic preparation of the left jugular fossa, placing an intravenous catheter, coupling an extension tube filled with heparinised saline solution. Each exercise test lasted for 28 minutes. It was run on a high-speed treadmill and consisted of incremental velocities to the maximum speed of 10 m/s of gallop (Table 1).

Table 1. Protocol of exercise test on a high-speed treadmill.

Speed (m/s)	Duration (minutes)	Inclination (%)	Gait
2.0	10	0	walk
4.0	2	6	trot
5.0	1	6	gallop
6.0	1	6	gallop
7.0	1	6	gallop
8.0	1	6	gallop
9.0	1	6	gallop
10.0	1	6	gallop
2.0	10	0	walk

Blood samples were obtained from the jugular vein, in syringes and immediately transferred to vacuum tubes containing sodium fluoride to determine plasma lactate concentrations. Blood samples were collected during the final 15 seconds of each speed. Plasma lactate concentrations were measured with a commercial reagent kit using a spectrophotometer.

Estimates of the velocity at which plasma lactate concentration reached 2 mmol/l (V_{LA2}) and 4 mmol/l (V_{LA4}) were obtained by exponential regression of the data, using the results of the lactate concentrations for each step. Statistical analysis was performed using descriptive statistics and the Student t-test for unpaired samples to compare the results before and after 22 weeks of the eventing season.

Results and discussion

Mean plasma lactate values of Brazilian Sport Horses training for eventing competitions during the exercise tests before and after the competitive season are shown in Table 2. There was an increase of plasma lactate values during the incremental speed peaking at 10 m/s. The increase of the plasma lactate concentration during the exercise test at the end of the competition season seemed to be higher than at the beginning (Table 2). But no significant difference ($P > 0.05$) was

Table 2. Plasma lactate concentration (mmol/l) of Brazilian Sport Horses before and after 22 weeks of an eventing season (mean ± standard deviation).

Speed during steps (m/s)	Exercise test at the start of competitive season	Exercise test after 22 weeks of competitive season
2.0	0.68±0.32	0.55±0.29
4.0	0.51±0.26	0.47±0.22
5.0	0.69±0.33	0.64±0.33
6.0	1.01±0.70	1.14±0.91
7.0	1.77±0.97	2.05±1.34
8.0	2.91±1.15	3.42±1.83
9.0	4.97±1.72	5.25±1.97
10.0	6.83±1.68	7.53±2.63
12.0	9.75±2.55	10.6±3.27

Table 3. Speed (m/s) when Brazilian Sport Horses training for eventing competitions reached a concentration of 2.0 mmol/l (V_{LA2}) and 4.0 mmol/l (V_{LA4}) of plasma lactate before and after 22 weeks of an eventing season (mean ± standard deviation (SD)).

Horse	Exercise test at the start of competitive season		Exercise test after 22 weeks of competitive season	
	V_{LA2}	V_{LA4}	V_{LA2}	V_{LA4}
1	4.94	7.07	3.20	5.56
2	6.95	8.34	6.96	8.42
3	6.83	8.25	7.05	8.58
4	7.06	8.06	7.22	8.53
5	7.23	8.58	5.31	6.90
6	5.33	7.08	6.36	7.47
7	6.64	7.99	6.68	7.82
Mean ± SD	6.43±0.91	7.91±0.60	6.11±1.43	7.61±1.10

found in the plasma lactate concentration behaviour before and after 22 weeks of an eventing season.

Individual and mean values for V_{LA2} and V_{LA4} of Brazilian Sport Horses during the exercise tests are shown in Table 3.

Mean V_{LA2} and V_{LA4} of the horses were lower 22 weeks after starting the competitive eventing season compared to the values at the beginning of the season but the difference was not significant ($P>0.05$). The performance of the horses during their eventing competitions was satisfactory for riders and trainers. Changes in the training program could be introduced with the aim of increasing V_{LA2} and V_{LA4} values of the horses to eventually improve performance too.

References

Davie, A.J and Evans, D.L., 2000. Blood lactate responses to submaximal field exercise tests in Thoroughbred horses. Veterinary Journal 159: 252-258.

Lindner, A., 2000. Use of blood biochemistry for positive performance diagnosis of sports horses in practice. Revue du Médecine Véterinaire 151: 611-618.

Lindner, A. and Boffi, F.M., 2007. Pruebas de ejercicio. In: Boffi, F.M. (ed.). Fisiologia del ejercicio en equinos. Editorial Interamerica, Buenos Aires, Argentina, pp. 243-254.

Marlin, D.J., Schroter, R.C., Mills, P.C., White, S.L., Maykuth, P.L., Votion, D. and Waran, N., 2001. Performance of acclimatized European horses in a modified one star three-day event in heat and humidity. Journal of Equine Veterinary Science 21: 341-350.

Snow, D.H. and Valberg, S.J., 1994. Muscle anatomy, physiology and adaptations to exercise and training. In: Hodgson, D.R. and Rose, R.J. (eds.). The athletic horse: principles and practice of equine sports medicine. WB Saunders, Philadelphia, PA, USA, pp. 145-179.

11. Effect of training for eventing on young Brazilian Sport Horses

F. Gomes Ferreira Padilha[1*], A.C. Tavares Miranda[2], A. Machado de Andrade[2], F. Queiroz de Almeida[2] and A.M. Reis Ferreira[1,3]

[1]Programa de Pós Graduação em Clínica e Reprodução Animal, Universidade Federal Fluminense, Brazil; [2]Universidade Federal Rural do Rio de Janeiro, Brazil; [3]Setor de Anatomia Patológica Veterinária, Universidade Federal Fluminense, Brazil; felipe_padilha@yahoo.com.br

Take home message

Morphological traits, body composition parameters, running duration at submaximal speed and blood plasma biochemical variables did not differ between 4- and 5-year-old Brazilian Sport Horses in training for eventing.

Keywords: biochemistry, blood, body weight, body fat, duration, enzymes, exercise test, morphology

Introduction

Brazilian Sport Horses were formed under the influence of horses of different breeds leading to their great genetic variability (Dias *et al.*, 2000) to obtain horses for different equestrian sports (SBBCH, 2015). The Brazilian Sport Horses are submitted to an intense exercise routine that can lead to changes in their conformation, body condition and to injuries if they are not adapted appropriately to this routine. The aim of this work was to evaluate the effect of eventing training on morphological traits, body composition, running duration at submaximal speed and blood plasma biochemical variables of 4- and 5-year-old Brazilian Sport Horses.

Materials and methods

The experiment was carried out at the Horse´s Performance Evaluation Laboratory (LADEq), located at the Brazilian Army Cavalry School, Rio de Janeiro, Brazil. Five 4-year old and six 5-year old Brazilian Sport

Horses were used. They were in training for eventing. Morphological traits, body weight, fat thickness, muscle mass and parameters derived from these variables, performance on a high speed treadmill and blood plasma biochemical variables were determined. The horses were fed with coastcross hay (*Cynodon dactylon*) and commercial concentrate, 50 g of mineral salt, and had free access to water. Their training program before measurements lasted for 9 months and 1 year 9 months long for the 4- and 5-year olds, respectively. Horses were exercised 5 days a week during 60 minutes. Exercise included flatwork, aerobic conditioning and jumping on both track and natural obstacles.

Evaluation of the morphological traits was performed according to Pinto *et al.* (2008). The horses were weighed on a mechanical scale. The measurement of rump fat layer was made by determining the thickness of adipose tissue of the muscle *gluteus medius* through ultrasound. The equation used to calculate the percentage of body fat was established by Kane *et al.* (1987):

% body fat = 2.47 + 5.47 (fat layer in cm).

The calculation of fat mass (in kg) of the horses was established by multiplying the weight of the animal by the percentage of body fat and the calculation of the fat free mass (in kg) was established by subtracting the fat mass of the horse's weight.

The performance was evaluated by an incremental speed test on a high-speed treadmill, exercising the horses until fatigue was declared (Table 1). Blood samples were obtained from the jugular vein in 10 ml tubes without anticoagulant. A 48 h resting period before blood sampling was respected to avoid an influence of exercise on the results. All data were measured at the end of the training season. Descriptive statistics were used and the Student t-test for unpaired samples to compare the groups.

Results and discussion

The morphological traits of young Brazilian Sport Horses in training for eventing competitions are shown in Table 2. There were no differences between groups.

Table 1. Incremental speed test protocol performed on a high-speed treadmill (adapted from Courouce-Malblanc and Hodgson, 2014).

Step	Duration (minutes)	Speed (m/s)	Gait	Inclination (%)
Warm-up	2	1.7	walk	0
Warm-up	4	4.0	trot	0
Warm-up	4	4.0	trot	3
Gallop	1	5.0	gallop	3
Gallop	1	6.0	gallop	3
Gallop	1	7.0	gallop	3
Gallop	No set time	8.0	gallop	3
Recovery	10	1.7	walk	0

Table 2. Morphological measurements of 4- and 5-year old Brazilian Sport Horses training for eventing (mean ± standard deviation).

Morphological variables	4-year olds	5-year olds
Withers height (m)	1.60±0.04	1.62±0.02
Height at croup (m)	1.62±0.02	1.63±0.02
Distance from the withers to the sternum (m)	0.69±0.01	0.69±0.02
Body length (m)	1.60±0.04	1.62±0.05
Length of croup (m)	0.53±0.02	0.52±0.03
Width of chest (m)	0.43±0.02	0.42±0.01
Width of croup (m)	0.55±0.01	0.55±0.03
Distance from the elbow to the ground (m)	0.92±0.02	0.92±0.03
Distance from the sternum to the ground (m)	0.86±0.02	0.86±0.02
Thoracic perimeter (m)	1.83±0.02	1.84±0.04

The weight, fat layer, percentage of body fat, fat mass and fat free mass of young Brazilian Sport Horses in training for eventing are shown in Table 3. Significant differences between groups were not observed.

The exercise duration at a speed of 8.0 m/s on the high-speed treadmill did not differ between 4- and 5-year old horses (267 ± 87

Table 3. Bodyweight, fat layer, percentage of body fat, fat mass and fat free mass of 4- and 5-year old Brazilian Sport Horses training for eventing (mean ± standard deviation).

Parameters	4-year-olds	5-year-olds
Body weight (kg)	486±40	506±21
Fat layer (cm)	0.49±0.24	0.48±0.24
Body fat (%)	5.16±1.30	5.10±1.34
Fat mass (kg)	25.3±7.61	25.9±7.16
Fat free mass (kg)	461±35	480±19

and 274 ± 76 seconds, respectively). Table 4 shows the values of blood plasma biochemical variables used in the evaluation of young Brazilian Sport Horses in training for eventing. Differences between age groups were not found.

There were no significant differences between 4- and 5-year-old Brazilian Sport Horses indicating that the training program did not improve fitness and based on the blood plasma biochemical variables it neither harmed the horses.

Table 4. Blood plasma biochemical variables of 4- and 5-year-old Brazilian Sport Horses training for eventing (mean ± standard deviation).

Variables[1]	4-year olds	5-year olds	Reference range[2]
AST (U/l)	286±54	307±104	150-400
CK (U/l)	158±19	180±26	100-300
Urea (mg/dl)	32.0±10.8	26.7±4.23	24-48
Creatinine (mg/dl)	1.43±0.15	1.44±0.18	1.1-1.8
GGT (U/l)	12.8±2.77	11.7±2.58	10-40
Albumin (g/dl)	2.83±0.10	2.89±0.21	2.6-3.8
Calcium (mg/dl)	13.3±0.38	13.2±0.81	10.8-13.2

[1] AST = aspartate aminotransferase; CK = creatine kinase; GGT = gamma-glutamyl transpeptidase.
[2] Reference values according to McGowan and Hodgson (2014).

References

Couroucé-Malblanc, A., and Hodgson D.R., 2014. Muscle anatomy, physiology, and adaptations to exercise and training. In: Hodgson, D.R., McKeever, K.H. and McGowan, C.M. (eds.) The athletic horse: principles and practice of equine sports medicine. Elsevier Saunders, St. Louis, MO, USA, pp. 366-378.

Dias, I.M.G., Bergmann, J.A.G., Rezende, A.C.C. and Castro, G.H.F, 2000. Formação e estrutura populacional do equino Brasileiro de Hipismo. Arquivo Brasileiro de Medicina Veterinária e Zootecnia 52: 647-654.

Kane, R.A., Fisher, M., Parrett, D. and Lawrence L.M., 1987. Estimating fatness in horses. In: Proceedings of the 10th Equine Nutrition and Physiology Symposium, Fort Collins, CO, USA, pp. 127-131.

McGowan, C.M. and Hodgson, D.R., 2014. Hematology and Biochemistry. In: Hodgson, D.R., McKeever, K.H. and McGowan, C.M. (eds.) The athletic horse: principles and practice of equine sports medicine. Elsevier Saunders, St. Louis, MO, USA, pp. 56-68.

Pinto, L.F.B., Almeida, F.Q., Quirino, C.R., Azevedo, P.C.N., Cabral, G.C., Santos, E.M. and Corassa, A., 2008. Evaluation of the sexual dimorphism in Mangalarga Marchador horses using discriminant analysis. Livestock Science 119: 161-166.

Stud Book Brasileiro do Cavalo de Hipismo (SBBCH), 2015. Regulamento. Available at: http://tinyurl.com/pk5efzw.

12. Effect of aleurone supplementation on postprandial glucose and insulin response in horses

C. Delesalle[1]*, A. Popovic[1], P. Hespel[2], J.E. de Oliveira[3], L. Duchateau[1], L. Verdegaal[4] and M. de Bruijn[5]

[1]Department of Comparative Physiology and Biometrics, Faculty of Veterinary Medicine, Ghent University, Belgium; [2]Bakala Academy, Athletic Performance Center, Leuven University, Belgium; [3]Cargill Research and Development Centre Europe, Havenstraat 84, 1800 Vilvoorde, Belgium; [4]School of Animal and Veterinary Science, University of Adelaide, Australia; [5]Wolvega Equine Hospital, Stellingenweg 10, 8474 EA Oldeholtpade, the Netherlands; catherine.delesalle@ugent.be

Take home message

Aleurone supplementation modulates energy metabolism in sports horses.

Keywords: energy, feeding, metabolism, nutrition, sport

Introduction

Aleurone, is thought to be responsible for the beneficial health effects of whole wheat products (Brouns et al., 2010, 2012). Aleurone is particularly rich in nutrients and bioactive phytochemicals such as antioxidants (e.g. ferulic acid), osmolytes (e.g. betaïne), vitamins (e.g. thiamin), essential aminoacids (e.g. lysine) and minerals (Buri et al., 2004). Studies report beneficial effects of aleurone on 5 main areas: (1) reduction of oxidative stress; (2) positive immunomodulatory effects; (3) energy management; (4) digestive health; and (5) vitamin and mineral stores (Brouns et al., 2012). To date, aleurone-related research has been performed either in vitro or in rodent models focusing on certain pathological conditions such as obesity. However, there is an increasing interest to evaluate the effect of aleurone in

A. Lindner (ed.) **Applied equine nutrition and training (ENUTRACO 2015)**
DOI 10.3920/978-90-8686-818-6_12, © Wageningen Academic Publishers 2015

healthy subjects, both human and animals. The bioavailability of the key components of the aleurone fraction depends on how good the organism succeeds in releasing them from the arabinoxylan containing fibre food matrix (Anson *et al.*, 2009). Before absorption into the circulation can take place, they need to be released from the tissue matrix either by intestinal mucosal enzymes or by the intestinal bacterial enzymes. It is expected in horses that fermentation by gut flora can greatly influence oral bioavailability of aleurone components in a positive way.

The current study specifically focused on postprandial glucose and insulin response in trotter horses at rest, fed concentrate feed with and without aleurone supplementation. The objective of the current study was to obtain a better insight into metabolism and pharmacokinetics of aleurone components on postprandial glycemic and insulin profiles in horses not subjected to training stress (Apicella *et al.*, 2013; Price *et al.*, 2010; Yde *et al.*, 2012).

Sports horses are often fed concentrate diets containing high soluble carbohydrate concentrations. It is known that these diets are improper for horses sensitive to pronounced changes in blood glucose levels, because of their reduced insulin sensitivity. Also in humans the negative effects of increased insulin resistance are well known (Lewitt *et al.*, 2014). Insulin promotes anabolic (storage) and inhibits catabolic (breakdown) processes. It promotes uptake and storage of glucose in muscle and fat cells and increases muscle glycogen storage efficiency. In human athletes, the beneficial effects of increased peripheral insulin sensitivity on performance capacity are well known (De Bock *et al.*, 2005).

Material and methods

An aleurone dosing trial using 8 healthy trotter horses not trained for competition and testing 4 different aleurone doses (50, 100, 200, and 400 g/day) during 10 consecutive weeks was applied. Two batches of concentrate feed were manufactured: (1) one pelletised blanco batch in which aleurone was replaced by wheat bran; and (2) a pelletised batch containing 20% aleurone. Both batches were mixed to achieve the proper aleurone dose. Each dose was fed during 7 consecutive days, followed by 1 week wash out during which only blanco concentrate feed was fed. Horses were fed a concentrate meal twice a day (8 am – aleurone enriched, and 8 pm). The one week doses were assigned to each of the 8 horses following a Latin square model. Horses were housed in individual boxes (14 m²) on wood shavings. They had free access to tab water and hay. The amount of hay consumed by each horse was recorded. The horses were turned out in paddocks two hours a day. Horses were customised to the blanco concentrate feed two weeks prior to the start of the study. Postprandial glycemic and insulin responses were monitored on day 7 of each week.

Blood was sampled when feeding started (T0) and every 30 min (4 h) and thereafter every 60 min (4 h) for glucose analysis (Na^+ fluoride tubes) and at T0 and every 10 min (1 h), thereafter every 30 min (4 h) for insulin analysis (heparin coated tubes). The data was organised as a replicated Latin square design for statistical analysis, with aleurone dose and time after feeding and their interaction as fixed effects. Statistical analysis included aleurone dose regression and curve analysis (time of peak value, peak value, and area under the curve).

Results

The interaction between aleurone dose and time was significant ($P < 0.05$) for both, glucose and insulin. Feeding aleurone delayed time of peak circulating glucose and insulin linearly as aleurone dose in the diet increased ($P < 0.05$). Glucose peak value and area under the curve were not affected by aleurone but insulin peak concentration in blood and area under the curve reduced linearly with increasing doses of aleurone in the diet ($P < 0.05$).

Conclusions

Aleurone supplementation has a beneficial effect on glucose and insulin response to concentrate meal uptake in horses. Glucose and insulin peak values are delayed and insulin peak values are lower in aleurone supplemented horses. More research is needed to evaluate possible performance enhancing effects of aleurone in horses in competition.

C. Delesalle et al.

References

Anson, N.M., Selinheimo, E., Havenaar, R., Aura, A.M., Mattila, I., Lehtinen, P., Bast, A., Poutanen, K. and Haenen, G.R., 2009. Bioprocessing of wheat bran improves *in vitro* bioaccessibility and colonic metabolism of phenolic compounds. Journal of Agricultural Food and Chemistry 57: 6148-6155.

Apicella, J.M., Lee, E.C., Bailey, B.L., Saenz, C., Anderson, J.M., Craig, S.A.S., Kraemer, W.J., Volek, J.S. and Maresh, C.M., 2013. Betaine supplementation enhances anabolic endocrine and Akt signaling in response to acute bouts of exercise. European Journal of Applied Physiology 113: 793-802.

Brouns, F., Adam-Perrot, A., Atwell, B. and Reding, W.V., 2010. Nutritional and technological aspects of wheat aleurone fiber: implications for use in food. In: Van der Kamp, J.W.M, Jones, J., McCleary, B. and Topping, D. (eds.) Dietary fiber: new frontiers for food and health. Wageningen Academic Publishers, Wageningen, the Netherlands, pp. 395-413.

Brouns, F., Hemery, Y., Price, R. and Anson, N.M., 2012. Wheat aleurone: separation, composition, health aspects, and potential food use. Critical Reviews in Food Science and Nutrition 52: 553-568.

Buri, R.C., Von Reding, W. and Gavin, M.H., 2004. Description and characterization of wheat aleurone. Cereal Foods World 49: 274-282.

De Bock, K., Richter, E.A., Rusell, A.P., Eijnde, B.O., Derave, W., Ramaekers, M., Koninckx, E., Léger, B., Verhaeghe, J. and Hespel, P., 2005. Exercise in the fasted state facilitates fibre type-specific intramyocellular lipid breakdown and stimulates glycogen resynthesis in humans. Journal of Physioly 564: 649-660.

Lewitt, M.S., Dent, M.S. and Hall, K., 2014. The insulin-like growth factor system in obesity, insulin resistance and type 2 diabetes mellitus. Journal of Clinical Medicine 3: 1561-1574.

Price, R.K., Keaveney, E.M., Hamill, L.L., Wallace, J.M.W., Ward, M., Ueland, P.M., McNulty, H., Strain, J.J., Parker, M.J. and Welch, R.W., 2010. Consumption of wheat aleurone-rich foods increases fasting plasma betaine and modestly decreases fasting homocysteine and LDL-cholesterol in adults. The Journal of Nutrition 140: 2153-2157.

Yde, C.C., Jansen, J.J., Theil, P.K., Bertram, H.C. and Knudsen, K.E.B., 2012. Different metabolic and absorption patterns of betaine in response to dietary intake of whole-wheat grain, wheat aleurone or rye aleurone in catheterized pigs. European Food Research and Technology 235: 939-949.

Related titles:

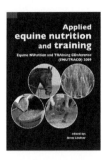

Applied equine nutrition

Equine NUtrition COnference (ENUCO) 2013

edited by: Arno Lindner

paperback ISBN 978-90-8686-240-5

e-book ISBN 978-90-8686-793-6

www.WageningenAcademic.com/ENUTRACO2013

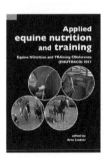

Applied equine nutrition and training

Equine NUtrition and TRAining COnference (ENUTRACO) 2011

edited by: Arno Lindner

paperback ISBN 978-90-8686-183-5

e-book ISBN 978-90-8686-740-0

www.WageningenAcademic.com/ENUTRACO2011

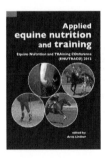

Applied equine nutrition and training

Equine NUtrition and TRAining COnference (ENUTRACO) 2009

edited by: Arno Lindner

paperback ISBN 978-90-8686-124-8

e-book ISBN 978-90-8686-669-4

www.WageningenAcademic.com/ENUTRACO2009

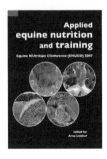

Applied equine nutrition and training

Equine NUtrition COnference (ENUCO) 2007

edited by: Arno Lindner

paperback ISBN 978-90-8686-040-1

e-book ISBN 978-90-8686-607-6

www.WageningenAcademic.com/ENUCO2007

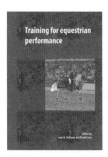

Training for equestrian performance
edited by: Jane Williams and David Evans
hardback ISBN 978-90-8686-258-0
www.WageningenAcademic.com/Equestrian

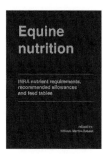

Equine nutrition
INRA nutrient requirements, recommended allowances and feed tables
edited by: William Martin-Rosset
hardback ISBN 978-90-8686-237-5
www.WageningenAcademic.com/EquineNutrition

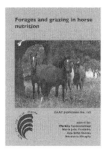

Forages and grazing in horse nutrition
EAAP Scientific Series, Volume 132
edited by: Markku Saastamoinen, Maria João Fradinho, Ana Sofia Santos and Nicoletta Miraglia
paperback ISBN 978-90-8686-200-9
e-book ISBN 978-90-8686-755-4
www.WageningenAcademic.com/EAAP132

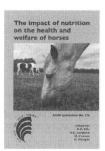

The impact of nutrition on the health and welfare of horses
EAAP Scientific Series, Volume 128
edited by: A. D. Ellis, A. C. Longland, M. Coenen and N. Miraglia
paperback ISBN 978-90-8686-155-2
e-book ISBN 978-90-8686-711-0
www.WageningenAcademic.com/EAAP128

Printed in the United States
by Baker & Taylor Publisher Services